DATE OF RETURN
UNLESS RECALLED BY LIBRARY

PLEASE TAKE GOOD CARE OF THIS BOOK

Dan Lipsker

Clinical Examination and Differential Diagnosis of Skin Lesions

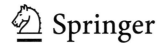 Springer

Dan Lipsker
Hôpital Universitaire de Strasbourg
Strasbourg
France

Translation from the French language edition 'Guide de l'examen clinique et du diagnostic en dermatologie' by Dan Lipsker, © Elsevier-Masson France, 2010; ISBN: 978-2294710308

ISBN 978-2-8178-0410-1   ISBN 978-2-8178-0411-8   (eBook)
DOI 10.1007/978-2-8178-0411-8
Springer Paris Heidelberg New York Dordrecht London

Library of Congress Control Number: 2013945861

Printed on acid-free paper

Springer is part of Springer Science+Business Media (www.springer.com)

Clinical Examination and Differential Diagnosis of Skin Lesions

To my children,
Louise and Gabriel.

Preface

This book has several objectives, the first being to guide the reader through a step-by-step training in dermatological examination. This essential approach is often neglected in medical studies and reference books which focus on teaching of diseases, especially their pathogenesis, prognosis, and treatment. Training in dermatological examination relies mainly on visual recognition and requires that the text be entirely focused on the description of lesions as well as being very richly illustrated. The first part of this book is exclusively dedicated to the identification of the primary lesions of the skin, which can be assimilated to the alphabet that needs to be learned to diagnose skin disorders. Another objective is to have access to a book which fills the gaps resulting from an overly rigid education during medical studies. Indeed, many students know perfectly the physiopathology of acne without knowing how to recognize the primary lesions characterizing this disorder. During their studies, many doctors have never observed the cardinal cutaneous signs of diseases which they will encounter during medical practice, such as neurofibromatosis, sarcoidosis, or mastocytosis. The same applies for benign and malignant skin tumors, although they are extremely frequent. Therefore, my wish was to illustrate diseases which doctors should have seen at least once. Again, for each of the selected diseases, emphasis was laid on the characteristic clinical aspects, both in the text and illustrations.

Finally, the last part of the work discusses the causes of various cutaneous signs (differential diagnosis) and naturally follows the first two parts. The reader will be provided with an overview of the scope of dermatological differential diagnosis, constituting a real help for diagnosis.

For Whom Is This Book Intended?

This book is mainly intended for medical students, general practitioners, internists, and training dermatologists. It will be their primary resource for the approach required to recognize primary lesions, as well as for annotated illustrations of the dermatologic expression of various diseases which they may encounter. The experienced dermatologist will find useful reminders of semantics and a chapter on differential diagnosis that can be helpful, should they get "stuck" on a diagnosis.

How to Read This Book?

Non-dermatologists are recommended to start by reading the first chapters devoted to semiology. The chapter on nosology can be covered by trying to describe each photograph before reading its caption. Dermatologists will skim through the chapters Semiology and Nosology and will refer to the chapter on Differential Diagnosis in the event of diagnostic difficulties.

I spent a long time looking for a book that meets these various goals. Having not found any and after lengthy hesitation, I decided to write one myself. I hope I have accomplished what I have set out to do and I wish an excellent reading to students and colleagues. I would be happy to receive any comment which would help improving a possible next edition. Kindly contact me by e-mail (dan.lipsker@chru-strasbourg.fr).

Strasbourg, France   Dan Lipsker

Thanks

Unless stated otherwise, all photographs come from the collection of the Dermatological Clinic of the University Hospital of Strasbourg.

I wish to thank M. Ph. Etcheverry of the central audiovisual and photography service, Faculty of Medicine, University of Strasbourg, for the editing of the digital photos.

Dan Lipsker

Contents

Introduction

A complete clinical examination should include an examination of the skin, the mucous membranes, the nails, the body hair, and the hair.

Such an examination helps to identify cutaneous signs associated with internal diseases, which are sometimes specific enough to allow diagnosis, and to recognize diseases specific to the skin. In most systemic diseases, more or less specific cutaneous signs can be present. For example, patients with diabetes may exhibit numerous skin manifestations, however rarely indicative of the disease (Fig. 1). On the other hand, in systemic lupus erythematosus, an autoimmune disease that can potentially affect all organs including the kidney, the heart, the serous membranes, and the central nervous system, cutaneous signs are often indicative of the disease (Fig. 2).

Cutaneous signs thus allow easy diagnosis of the disease due to their immediate visibility. This accessibility also easily enables the possibility of biopsies for clinicopathological correlation, in cases where diagnosis cannot be confirmed solely on clinical grounds. Histopathological confirmation of numerous diseases can therefore be obtained while avoiding biopsies of less accessible internal organs.

Systematic skin examination also enables the detection of disorders which are specific to the skin, in particular early-stage melanoma (Fig. 3), a dreadful skin cancer always fatal in advanced stages.

> Many diseases may include cutaneous signs that can sometimes help to reveal them. Because of the easy accessibility of skin for biopsy, a clinicopathological correlation is possible in almost any situation.

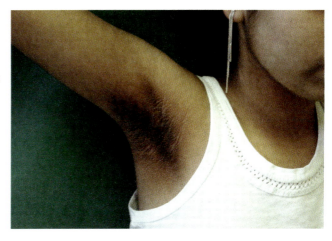

Fig. 1 Acanthosis nigricans. Brown and rough aspect of axillae, conferring a "dirty" appearance. This is acanthosis nigricans, often a marker of insulin resistance, as in the case of this young girl. When acanthosis nigricans is of recent onset and diffuse, and particularly circumoral and acral, it can be a paraneoplastic syndrome requiring to further investigate the possibility of cancer

Fig. 2 Lupus erythematosus. Red facial lesions that are indicative of an autoimmune disease called systemic lupus erythematosus. It is a symmetrical congestive erythema of the midface (in the shape of a butterfly) which partially spares the sun-protected areas of the nasolabial folds. Labial erosions can also be noted. This young woman has also developed severe renal impairment as well as pleurisy

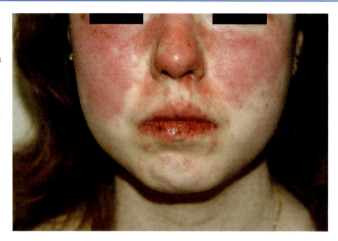

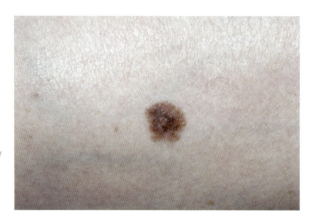

Fig. 3 Melanoma. Brown spot, irregularly colored: this is a melanoma, a skin cancer with poor prognosis. There is no effective treatment for advanced forms and only early diagnosis allows for recovery

Part I

Semiology

Clinical Examination and Approach to the Patient in Dermatology

Diagnosis of cutaneous lesions requires both history taking and physical examination. History taking must specify the circumstances of the onset and the course of the disease, as well as treatments applied and their effects. The starting date of the disorder and its initial location must be specified, as well as the ways in which the lesions spread and eventually change. The main cutaneous functional symptoms are pain and pruritus. The context in which lesions have appeared is often essential: associated extracutaneous signs, medications, comorbidities, immunodeficiencies, etc. Thus full history taking is often crucial, gathering all past history. Finally, given the large number of skin diseases related to the environment, targeted history taking should be carried out regarding lifestyle, professional and domestic backgrounds, and products that may have been applied and manipulated, in order not to miss, for example, the diagnosis of a contact dermatitis. Dermatological *physical examination* requires training. It is necessary to know how to recognize the primary lesions of the skin, their arrangement and/or configuration, and their distribution.

Primary lesions are the skin's response to aggressions and diseases. The term *elementary lesions,* which clearly reflects the fact that those lesions are the basic response patterns of the skin, is used in the French dermatologic literature. Every skin disorder can be described by means of its constitutive primary lesions. Therefore, a limited set of lesions describes all skin disorders. These lesions can thus be compared to the letters of the alphabet. Their combination produces syndromes.

The *arrangement* is the positioning of the various lesions relatively to each other. For example, they can form a line ("linear arrangement") (Fig. 1.1). In herpes, the different vesicles tend to group in clusters (Fig. 1.2).

Configuration indicates the shape of an isolated primary lesion. For example, a lesion can be annular (Fig. 1.3) or target-shaped (Fig. 1.4).

Distribution indicates the spread of the disease that is the parts of the body where the lesions are located. For example,

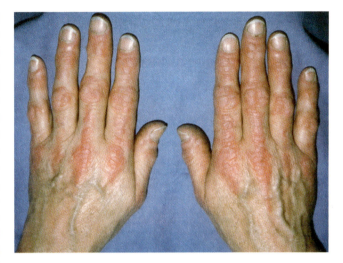

Fig. 1.1 Dermatomyositis. Linearity. Palpable linear erythema of the back of the hands. The general rule is that linearity results from the action of an external agent. Here, dermatomyositis is an exception to this rule since it is an endogenous disease which causes the linear erythema, extending from the back of the hand to the dorsal aspect of the fingers. Dermatomyositis is a serious disease affecting the skin, muscles, and sometimes the lungs, digestive tract, and other organs. Treatment is based on systemic corticosteroids sometimes combined with immunosuppressants

it may be a single, thus localized lesion, as is the case in tumors; it may also be a generalized eruption affecting the entire skin, for example, in certain drug reactions or virally induced eruptions.

In practice, two types of situations can be pointed out: common situations (acne, warts, etc.) or single lesions (tumors) and more complex situations. In the first case, it may be useful to quickly proceed to a physical examination. In all the other cases, it is preferable to begin with history taking since the precise history of the disease, the personal and family histories, and the review of systems provide essential and even indispensable information for proper diagnosis. Indeed, it must be borne in mind that almost all

D. Lipsker, *Clinical Examination and Differential Diagnosis of Skin Lesions,*
DOI 10.1007/978-2-8178-0411-8_1, © Springer-Verlag France 2013

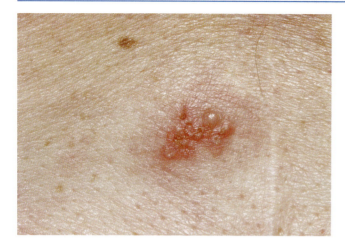

Fig. 1.2 Herpes. Herpetiformis. Several liquid lesions (called vesicles) on a *red* background and close to each other. In this example, the arrangement of these lesions is said to be herpetiform, since it is characteristic of herpesvirus infections. Two other signs characterizing vesicles of viral origin can be observed: the specific *gray* color and most importantly the central subsidence of several vesicles, called umbilication

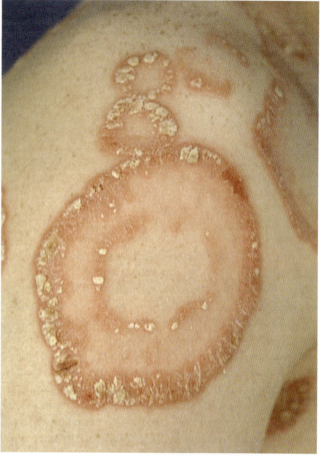

diseases can induce cutaneous manifestations, which can sometimes help reveal them. This implies taking into account the whole history and all other clinical signs (history taking and physical examination data) in making a diagnosis.

The reasoning mechanisms that allow making a diagnosis based on visual analysis are twofold:

- An analogical mechanism, where the physician recognizes a disease he has already observed
- An analytical mechanism, in which the physician recognizes one or more primary lesions with their distribution and/or configuration and/or arrangement and/or evolution enabling him to make one or more diagnoses, without necessarily having observed this dermatosis beforehand

It is necessary to keep in mind the following points:

- The semiological analysis of the cutaneous lesions must always be considered in the general context of the patient: his/her medical history, the complete history of his/her disease, other clinical signs, etc. Otherwise, there is high risk of either making a wrong diagnosis or ignoring the causality.
- One should avoid confusion between semiology (study of signs) and nosology (study of diseases). Papules, for example, have many causes including urticaria. Urticaria, for instance, corresponds to nosology since it can be the cutaneous expression of many different diseases. Urticaria can occur, for example, in a patient with thyroid dysfunction or as a result of drug allergy. Similarly with comedo, its identification requires a careful semiological approach. Interpretation is based on nosology

Fig.1.3 Psoriasis. Annularity. Red scaly lesions that form a ring in psoriasis. This is an annular configuration, i.e., a single lesion which extends centrifugally to produce this particular pattern. Psoriasis is a very common disease, affecting about 2 % of the world population

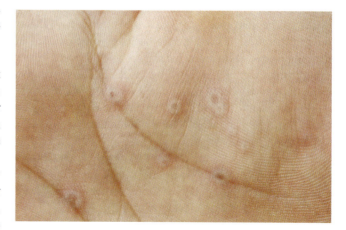

Fig.1.4 Erythema multiforme. Target-shaped. The target-shaped configuration consists in several concentric rings, characteristic of erythema multiforme. In erythema multiforme, an often parainfectious hypersensitivity reaction (particularly related to herpesvirus), this type of cutaneous lesions is associated with erosive mucosal injury which can sometimes be severe

since the causes of comedo are varied. The most common cause is acne; however, the following conditions may also be comedonal: follicular mucinosis and mycosis fungoides, lupus erythematosus, heliosis (Favre-Racouchot syndrome), follicular form of Darier's disease, drug eruption and intoxication (dioxin, amineptine, etc.), nevus comedonicus, facial papules occurring in certain B cell blood dyscrasias, etc.

Always list all the existing primary lesions, their configuration, arrangement and distribution, as well as their history. It is also necessary to specify the context in which these lesions appeared, the associated extracutaneous signs, and the history of the patient.

Physical Examination in Dermatology: Primary Lesions

The analysis of certain characteristics such as shape, size, surface, and color of a lesion has enabled the identification of "primary or elementary lesions" which represent the skin's response to various diseases and aggressions. All skin lesions are the result of the combination of one or several primary lesions, i.e., the most elementary lesions that can represent various skin diseases and may be used to describe them. In order to be classified as primary, a lesion must be easily identified from another without confusion. Primary lesions allow the description of all alterations of the skin. The combination of several of these lesions can produce actual syndromes. The primary lesions consist in an "alphabet" that the physician must learn to recognize in order to be able to describe and to diagnose a skin disease by inspecting, palpating, and folding the skin. Good lighting is essential.

First, it must be determined whether the lesion is *palpable*. Most of the time, a lesion is "obviously" palpable as it is physically elevated or depressed (Fig. 2.1); however, it must sometimes be brushed with the finger in order to feel any difference of consistency compared to adjacent skin. *Palpable lesions may be solid or contain fluid*. In other situations, the skin must be pinched between the thumb and forefinger in order to feel deeply any palpable formation. Palpation, folding, and stretching of the skin also enable to identify *changes in its consistency*. The skin may lack suppleness or even be too supple or too loose. During clinical examination, other elements such as *temperature and sensitivity* of lesions must also be evaluated.

Skin may become palpable due to an *alteration of its surface*. It is very important to determine whether a lesion is itself palpable since this is almost always due to an abnormality of the dermis or of deeper structures or simply to an alteration of the skin surface resulting from epidermal lesion (Fig. 2.2). Skin can also be palpable for both reasons.

Alterations of the skin surface are discussed in detail in Chap. 7. They are briefly presented here to explain the diagnostic approach. Skin surface is altered when

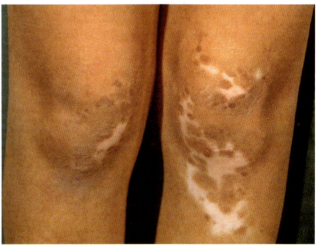

Fig. 2.2 Leukodermic macule. Piebaldism. The skin around the knee is either too fair (hypopigmented or leukodermic lesion) or too dark (hyperpigmented). However, these lesions are not palpable. These localized, impalpable, anomalies of skin color are called maculae. Here, they are a manifestation of piebaldism, a genetic disease. The geometric shape of the white lesions, their location on the knees, and the peripheral hyperpigmentation are all characteristic of this rare disease

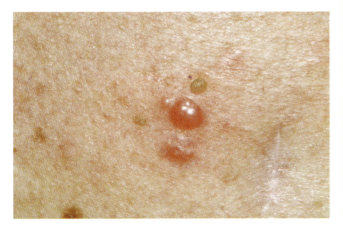

Fig. 2.1 Palpable lesions. Lymphoma, nevus, seborrheic keratosis. These are obviously "visually" palpable lesions as they are clearly raised. The *red* lesions are related to a cutaneous B cell lymphoma, while the brown ones are nevi and seborrheic keratoses, which are very common benign lesions. Also note the white depressed scar

D. Lipsker, *Clinical Examination and Differential Diagnosis of Skin Lesions*, DOI 10.1007/978-2-8178-0411-8_2, © Springer-Verlag France 2013

- *Thickened*, the skin, usually smooth, becomes rough (Fig. 2.3).
- *Thinned*, it becomes too thin and transparent (Fig. 2.4).
- *Absent*, causing oozing or bleeding (Fig. 2.5) and evolving towards a crust.
- *Interrupted or broken*, by a depression or orifice (Fig. 2.6).
- *Covered* with scales (Fig. 2.7) or crusts (Fig. 2.8.).
- *Raised* due to the presence of fluid, whether clear (Fig. 2.9), cloudy, or hemorrhagic.
- *Insensitive*, and cold, thus rapidly evolving into black necrosis (Fig. 2.10).

Alterations of the skin surface can occur on formerly healthy skin or may complicate the course of other primary lesions, in which case they can be used as adjectives to better describe them.

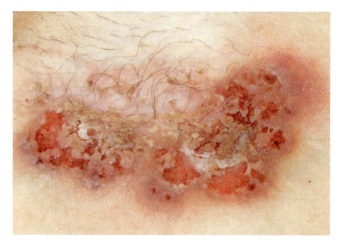

Fig. 2.5 Cribriform ulceration. Pyoderma gangrenosum. Skin defect: ulceration. Healing can also be observed as being cribriform, that is, by forming a screening that defines ulcerated areas by creating a network; this type of healing is highly characteristic of pyoderma gangrenosum, a neutrophilic inflammatory disease particularly associated with myeloid blood diseases and cryptogenic inflammatory diseases of the intestine

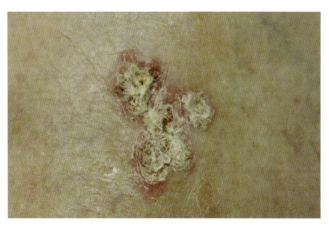

Fig. 2.3 Keratosis. Bowen's disease. This *red* lesion is covered with a highly adherent *yellow white* coating, rough to the touch, called keratosis. This example shows an in situ squamous cell carcinoma or Bowen's disease. Unlike scale (see Fig. 2.7), keratosis cannot be easily detached; forcefully pulling it off causes bleeding

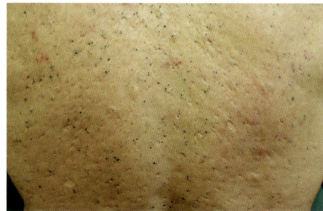

Fig. 2.6 Depression. Scar, comedo, acne. In this photograph, flattened cutaneous depressions may be noted that indicate a dermal atrophy due to scarring sequelae of severe acne, as well as numerous black dots corresponding to comedos. Comedo is an invagination of the skin surface filled with keratin while the epidermis is normally present, whereas it is absent in case of erosion or ulceration

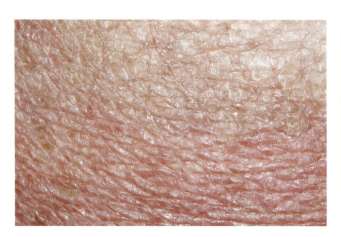

Fig. 2.4 Atrophy. Mycosis fungoides. The skin is thin, shiny, and wrinkled, being atrophic. It is also erythematous. In this patient, the skin atrophy results from a cutaneous T cell lymphoma called mycosis fungoides

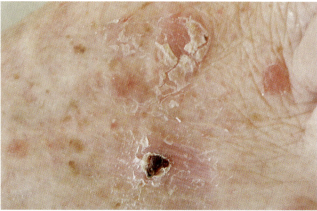

Fig. 2.7 Scale. The skin is red and covered with a coating which is easily removed (scales), unlike keratosis (cf. Fig. 2.3) which is adherent. One can also note the presence of a darker lesion, corresponding to a crust

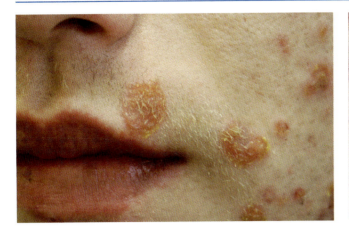

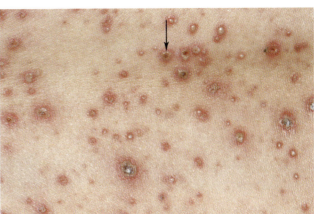

Fig. 2.8 Crusts. Impetigo. Grumous *yellow* lesions that may come off: these are crusts. In this example, the more or less rounded form of the lesions, their *yellow color* (honey-colored), and circumoral distribution enable diagnosis of impetigo. Impetigo is a skin infection caused by streptococci or staphylococci, often occurring on healthy skin of children and almost always on preexisting dermatoses in adults. Hence the aphorism "all impetigo occurring in adult is scabies until proven otherwise"

Fig. 2.11 Lesional dynamics. Varicella. This picture shows the lesional dynamics during varicella in which elements of different age groups coexist. The following can be seen: submillimeter-sized vesicles, the very initial lesions, vesicles on an erythematous background, pustules of variable sizes, and finally some pustules with a central depression (umbilication, *arrow*) and crusts

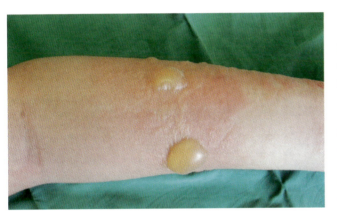

Fig. 2.9 Bulla. Eczema. In this photograph, the skin surface is elevated by a lesion filled with fluid, a bulla, measuring more than 1 cm. Note that this bulla is sited on a red skin (erythematous); it is a bullous contact dermatitis

Finally, it must be kept in mind that primary lesions can be progressive and change with time. For example, in urticaria, primary lesions are randomly distributed papules or plaques which are gathered in polycyclic figures and are of migratory and transient progression. In varicella (Fig. 2.11), primary lesions are vesicles with a cutaneomucosal distribution, bear no distinctive configuration, and progress towards umbilication and crusting. Also, in these two examples, progression is either intrinsic to the primary lesion (e.g., transiency of an edematous papule) or progressing towards a secondary lesion (e.g., evolution of a viral vesicle into an umbilicated pustule and a crust). The chronology of primary lesions is therefore important. For primary lesions, the following concepts must be specified: acuity, chronicity, and simultaneity of two lesions; asynchrony of two or three lesions; and their progression or regression over time.

An identification algorithm of primary lesions is proposed on Fig. 2.12 and on the book cover.

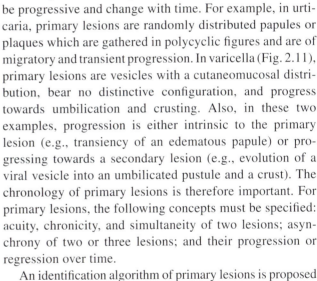

Fig. 2.10 Necrosis. Black necrosis area, well circumscribed and sharply delineated from the adjacent healthy skin by an eliminating groove. Necrosis reflects cutaneous ischemia, consisting in a devitalized and insensitive skin

Always observe, palpate, and fold the skin.

If the lesion is palpable, its content can be solid or liquid. The skin surface can be normal or altered. These elements determine the diagnostic process.

If the lesion is not palpable, it is then a localized or diffused modification of the color or transparency of the skin.

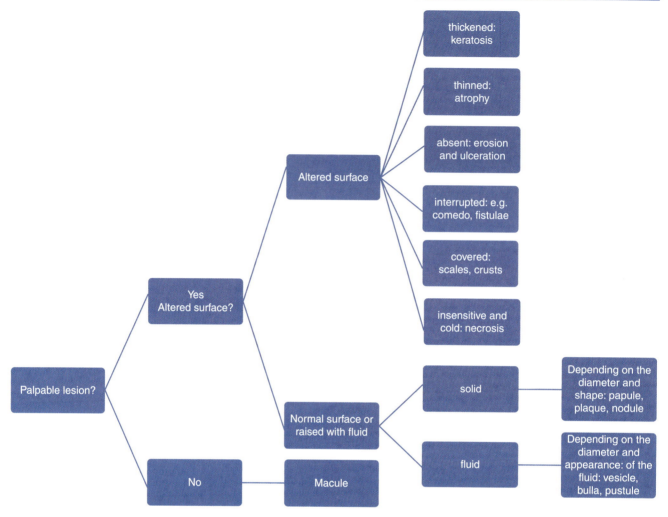

Fig. 2.12 Algorithm for the identification of the main primary lesions

Flat Lesions

3.1 Macule

When a lesion is not palpable, it becomes apparent because of localized skin discoloration. These lesions are usually called macules when they measure less than 2 cm and patches when they are larger. This distinction between macules and patches, based on diameter, has no practical interest and therefore the term macule will be used to refer to localized changes in skin color, regardless of size. Macules are classified according to color.

A macule can result from an anomaly residing exclusively in the epidermis (e.g., vitiligo, lentigine: Figs. 3.1 and 3.2), in the dermis (e.g., petechia, drug-induced maculopapular exanthema: Fig. 3.3), or in the epidermis and the dermis (e.g., postinflammatory hyperpigmentation: Fig. 3.4). Macules can be classified according to their color and reaction to glass test (diascopy).

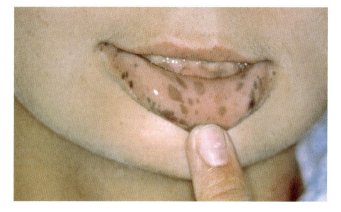

Fig. 3.2 Pigmented macules. Lentigo. Multiple brown macules of the lips. This is a case of mucosal lentigo. When macules are numerous and localized on the lips, they can be markers for Peutz-Jeghers syndrome, a diagnosis that should then be considered (see Chap. 15). In this syndrome, lentigines are associated with gastrointestinal polyposis as well as an increased risk of some non-gastrointestinal cancers

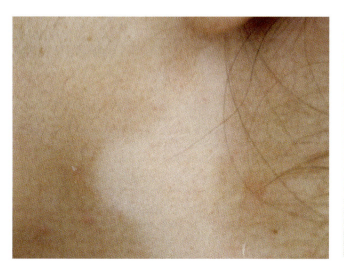

Fig. 3.1 White macule. Vitiligo. A macule is a localized anomaly of the color or transparency of the skin. By definition, a macule is not palpable. This example is a white macule observed in vitiligo. Vitiligo causes depigmentation of the skin. This autoimmune disorder of unknown origin can sometimes be associated with other autoimmune disorders such as thyroiditis or Biermer's disease. Note that the vellus hair present on the leukodermic macule in this patient is also depigmented

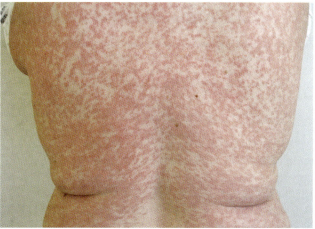

Fig. 3.3 Maculopapular exanthema. Skin reaction after use of dextropropoxyphene. Exanthema indicates the rapid and eruptive onset of circumscribed skin lesions on almost the entire integument. The lesions may be confluent, as shown in this example. These are macules, papules, and red plaques. In this example, the eruption was due to an analgesic allergy ("cutaneous drug reaction"). This type of drug reaction is common (see Chap. 12). Lesions disappear within a few days after discontinuation of the drug

D. Lipsker, *Clinical Examination and Differential Diagnosis of Skin Lesions*,
DOI 10.1007/978-2-8178-0411-8_3, © Springer-Verlag France 2013

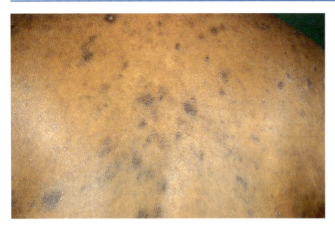

Fig. 3.4 Postinflammatory macules of the back. Lichen (planus). Brown pigmented macules of strong or mild coloration, resulting from lichen. According to the phototype of the individual, many inflammatory dermatoses can leave temporary or longer-lasting sequelae which are either hypopigmented ("postinflammatory hypopigmentation") or hyperpigmented ("postinflammatory hyperpigmentation"). Because they do not have any histopathological specificity, a retrospective diagnosis cannot be made

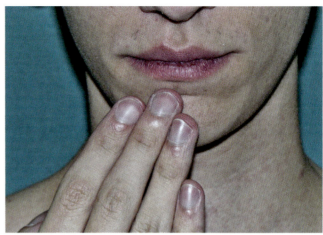

Fig. 3.6 Cyanosis in the context of hepatopulmonary syndrome. Bluish aspect of the lips and extremities, typical of a central cyanosis. Central cyanosis reflects a significant reduction in the arterial oxygen saturation (at least 2–3 g deoxyhemoglobin/100 mL), whereas peripheral cyanosis is the result of excessive extraction of oxygen in peripheral tissues, thus explaining its location at the extremities and the nose and the sparing of mucous membranes

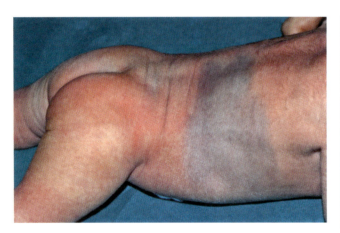

Fig. 3.5 Cerulodermic macule. Mongolian spot. Extended bluish-gray macule of several centimeters in a newborn. These lesions, called Mongolian spots, are common among newborns of Asian and North African origin. They have no special implication and usually regress with time

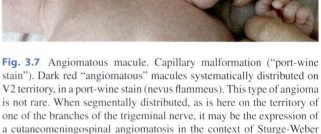

Fig. 3.7 Angiomatous macule. Capillary malformation ("port-wine stain"). Dark red "angiomatous" macules systematically distributed on V2 territory, in a port-wine stain (nevus flammeus). This type of angioma is not rare. When segmentally distributed, as is here on the territory of one of the branches of the trigeminal nerve, it may be the expression of a cutaneomeningospinal angiomatosis in the context of Sturge-Weber syndrome. This is especially true if sited on the V1 territory

Discolored (or dyschromic) macules can be white (e.g., vitiligo: Fig. 3.1), pigmented (e.g., lentigo: Fig. 3.2), bluish-gray (e.g., Mongolian spot: Fig. 3.5), or yellow (e.g., planar xanthoma).

The red macules deserve special mention due to their semiological features and their prevalence. They can be caused by active or passive vasodilation (e.g., exanthema, cyanosis: Figs. 3.3 and 3.6) or by intravascular blood accumulation (e.g., angioma: Fig. 3.7). They disappear on diascopy as opposed to purpuric macules which result from extravascular deposits of red blood cells and which persist on diascopy (Fig. 3.8).

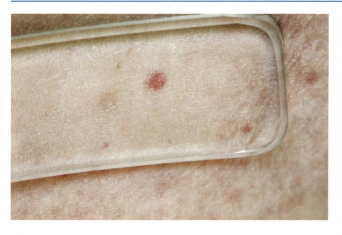

Fig. 3.8 Purpuric macule. Diascopy. Red macule not disappearing when pressure is applied on the skin with a transparent glass forcing out blood from the vessels (diascopy technique): It is therefore purpura, resulting from an intracutaneous hemorrhage; red blood cells being no longer in the vessels, the color persists on diascopy

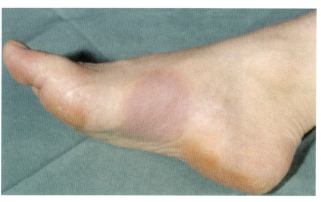

Fig. 3.9 Medioplantar erythematous macule. Fixed drug eruption. Fixed drug eruption is a cutaneous reaction to a drug occurring repeatedly in the same location each time the drug is taken and progressing towards a (postinflammatory) pigmentation sequela

3.2 Erythema

Erythema is a localized or diffuse redness (Fig. 3.9) of the skin which disappears on diascopy. It is either permanent or paroxysmal, sometimes reticulated (livedo) (Fig. 3.10) and at other times bluish (erythrocyanosis). Its color varies from pale pink to dark red. Erythema is often associated with desquamation, thus producing erythematosquamous lesions (see Fig. 2.7).

Diffuse erythema is often the combination of flat lesions and palpable lesions (papules and/or plaques), resulting in a maculopapular exanthema if of sudden onset (Fig. 3.3). Exanthema which consists of red macules and of barely palpable red lesions which tend to merge while leaving intervals of unaffected skin is referred to as morbilliform exanthema. Pink or red well-individualized lesions of generally less than 2 cm are referred to as roseola. In case of intense and diffuse redness, merging without leaving intervals of unaffected skin and presenting a grainy feel on palpation, it is referred to as scarlatiniform exanthema. Finally, a diffuse erythema of prolonged progression is called erythroderma, if affecting 90 % or more of the body surface area, immediately or very quickly accompanied by exfoliation and often by general symptoms such as fever and chills (Fig. 3.11).

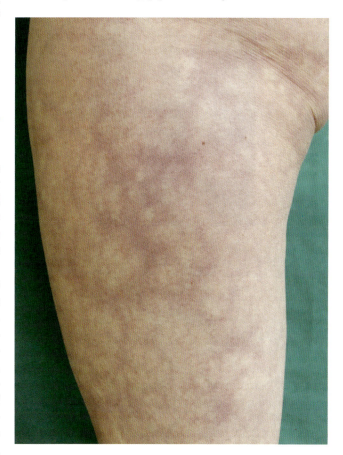

Fig. 3.10 Livedo. A netlike erythema. The livedo shown here is pathological. It is different from the physiological livedo (see Fig. 22.1) which is common particularly in newborns and which presents fine, regular, and closed meshes. In this patient, the meshes are thick (>1 cm) and highly purplish and are not always closed. This type of livedo indicates a thrombotic vasculopathy. The livedo in this example is symptomatic of a Sneddon's syndrome, where it is associated with iterative cerebral ischemic strokes

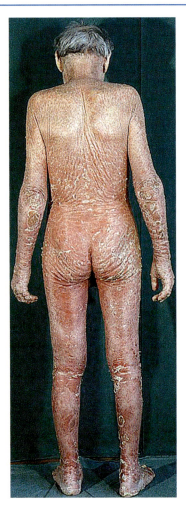

millimeters long that disappear easily on diascopy: They are known as telangiectases (Fig. 3.12). Some other primary lesions can also become telangiectatic (e.g., jugal erythema in rosacea or the tumoral nodule of basal cell carcinoma).

3.5   Poikiloderma

Poikiloderma is defined by the association of cutaneous atrophy, reticular pigmentation, and telangiectases (Fig. 3.13). Although poikiloderma is classically described as a primary lesion, it is more related to a syndrome (intricate lesions; see further) as it is a combination of several primary lesions.

3.6   Purpura

Purpura is permanent redness of the skin which does not disappear on diascopy, thus indicating an intracutaneous hemorrhage. Purpura may be circumscribed or widespread; it can be of varying tones ranging from red to blue, green, and yellow (Fig. 3.14) and may leave on its wake a temporary or lasting brown sequela. The following are known as:

- Petechiae, small-sized purpuric lesions.
- Vibices, more or less broad and elongated linear purpuric striae.
- Ecchymoses, extended purpuric patches with more or less irregular outlines, often of varying coloration (Fig. 3.14).

Purpura can sometimes be palpable (purpuric papule) (Fig. 3.15). If so, it is the manifestation of an inflammation of the vascular walls, i.e., vasculitis. Other clinical relevant varieties of purpura (i.e., retiform purpura) are described in the clinicopathological correlation section at the end of this chapter and in Chap. 23. Some lesions are red and do not or barely disappear on diascopy, but do not correspond to purpura. They are burgundy red in color and any experienced clinician will readily recognize their angiomatous nature (Fig. 3.7). This particular color can be related to macules but more often to infiltrate lesions (plaques). These lesions are described as angiomatous.

Fig. 3.11 Erythroderma. Psoriasis. This is a lasting erythema (≥15 days) rapidly evolving towards desquamation. Independently of its cause, erythroderma can be followed by life-threatening failure of the thermoregulatory and biological envelope functions of the skin

3.3   Cyanosis

Cyanosis corresponds to a change in skin color to purplish blue, with lowering of the temperature of extremities and mucous membranes when of central origin (Fig. 3.6).

3.4   Telangiectases

Certain non-palpable red lesions correspond to a permanent dilation of small vessels in the superficial dermis. They take the form of small sinuous lines of a few

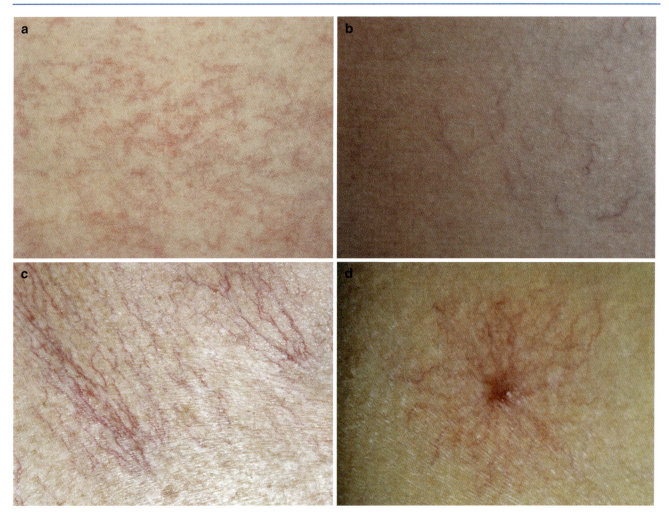

Fig. 3.12 Telangiectases (**a**, **b**, **c**, **d**). Four examples of telangiectases. In telangiectases, the small super ficial blood vessels become apparent, because they are permanently dilated. They can be isolated as shown in this figure or associated with other primary lesions. Telangiectases can be very thin and super ficial with diameters ≤0.5 mm (red telangiectases, **a**) or can be deeper located in the dermis with diameters greater than 1–2 mm (**b**, **c**). When deeper located, they are either blue telangiectases (0.5–1 mm) or phlebectases (≥1 mm). Finally, the last figure shows telangiectases which seem to converge towards a millimeter-wide central red papule (**d**). The pressure from this central papule, which corresponds to an afferent arteriole, allows emptying the telangiectases: this is a vascular spider (or spider nevus or nevus araneus)

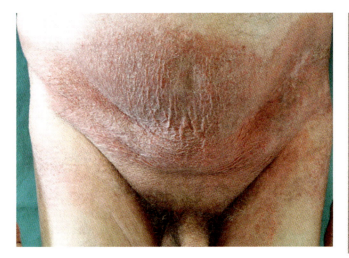

Fig. 3.13 Poikiloderma. Cutaneous T cell lymphoma. Widely spread poikiloderma in the abdominopelvic area. It is the resulting combination of three primary lesions: atrophy, very marked here and appearing as a thin and wrinkled skin; dyschromia, combining hypo- and hyperpigmented areas; and telangiectases

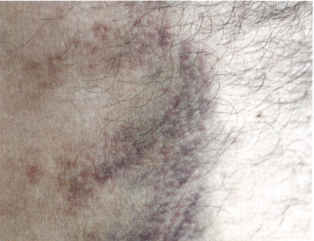

Fig. 3.14 Ecchymosis. Characteristic combinations of different colorations typical of purpura: red, purple, blue, green, yellow, and brown. This example shows a posttraumatic ecchymosis

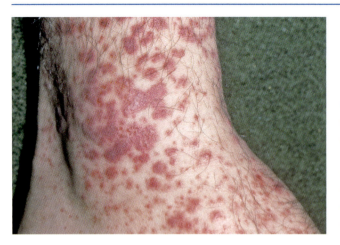

Fig. 3.15 Palpable purpura. Vasculitis. Palpable purpura or purpuric papule. A palpable purpura is usually the expression of a vasculitis, i.e., an inflammation of the vascular walls. Vasculitis can affect the skin as well as other organs such as the kidneys, the digestive tract, and the joints

Fig. 3.16 Shiny and leukodermic atrophic macule. Lichen sclerosus. White lesion (leukodermic) of wrinkled surface, indicating a thinned and atrophic epidermis, typical of lichen sclerosus. When its site is the genital area, as is generally the case, lichen sclerosus can become cancerous, thus justifying a long-term treatment and follow-up

3.7   Atrophic Macule

A non-palpable lesion can sometimes maintain a natural or white color but may become visible due to an unusual transparency of the skin. The underlying vessels thus become apparent as the skin becomes smooth and finely wrinkled, resembling "cigarette paper": It then constitutes an atrophic macule (Fig. 3.16).

As with all primary lesions, alterations of the surface may appear on a macule which then becomes palpable, hence producing a combination of primary lesions referred to as intricate lesions. For instance, in the course of pityriasis versicolor, primary lesions are sand-colored macule, primarily or mostly secondarily squamous, often confluent and distributed over the upper half of the trunk.

3.8   Clinicopathological Correlations: Mechanisms

3.8.1   Erythema and Angioma

Erythema indicates a disorder of the dermis and is often the result of a dilatation of dermal vessels or of a perivascular cellular infiltrate. The noninflammatory dilation of dermal vessels is responsible for permanent erythema, which hardly disappears on diascopy. This is the case with angiomas. On the other hand, erythema resulting from a perivascular inflammatory lymphocytic or neutrophilic infiltrate produces a redness that always clears easily under diascopy.

3.8.2   Purpura

It does not clear with diascopy because it is the clinical expression of an extravasation of red blood cells outside vessels. Certain types of clinical purpura display a particular histopathological picture:

- Non-infiltrated stellate or netlike purpura: often dark red and progressing towards necrosis, this indicates a thrombotic obliteration of dermal vessels as in the stages of disseminated intravascular coagulation, for example.
- Palpable purpura: generally a combination of purpura and erythema, due to an inflammation of the walls of dermal vessels called vasculitis.

3.8.3   Telangiectasia

A permanent dilation of postcapillary venules. Various types exist clinically and histopathologically.

3.8.4   Cyanosis

No histopathological expression. It is the consequence of intravascular stasis due to low hemoglobin. Cyanosis of central, cardiac, and pulmonary origins affects the extremities and mucous membranes, while peripheral cyanosis does not affect the mucous membranes.

3.8.5   Livedo

A netlike erythema. Its meshes usually reflect venous stasis in the area of an afferent cutaneous arteriole with decreased flow. In order to find the causative histopathological abnormality, multiple sections are required on a deep and large biopsy. Indeed, livedo can be due to the obliteration (multiple causes) of an afferent cutaneous arteriole possessing muscular walls and of diameter greater than

50 μm, located at the dermo-hypodermic junction or in the hypodermis.

3.8.6 Color of Macules

The color of macules gives an indication of their histogenesis and their potential causes.

3.8.6.1 Yellow (Xanthoderma)
It can be due to the alteration of the epidermis or dermis, thus resulting mostly from the following:
- Thickening of the stratum corneum producing a yellow keratosis
- Alteration of the connective tissue, particularly of elastic fibers (e.g., in the case of pseudoxanthoma elasticum) or of collagen bundles (e.g., in collagenic hamartomas)
- Abnormal deposits, particularly lipid deposit (e.g., xanthomas) or lipoprotein deposit (e.g., lipoproteinosis)
- Excessive deposit of carotene in the hypodermis and the stratum corneum, as well as elimination of the carotene pigments in the sebum, following hypercarotenemia
- Granulomatous or histiocytic cell infiltrate

3.8.6.2 White (Leukoderma)
It can be due to an epidermal alteration as well as a condition affecting the dermis. It is most often due to:
- A lack of melanin pigment, which can be caused by:
  - A decrease in the number of melanocytes or their complete disappearance (melanocytopenic hypomelanosis)
  - A defect in melanin synthesis or transfer (melanopenic hypomelanosis)
- A localized vasoconstriction: thus producing paleness
- Various mechanisms, not necessarily related to a pigment disorder:
  - Special keratosis as in warts or molluscum contagiosum
  - Tension exerted on the epidermis by the wall of a cyst, for example
  - Deposit of a white substance (e.g., cutaneous calcification)
  - Cutaneous sclerosis or hyalinization of collagen bundles as in morphea or lichen sclerosus and cutaneous infarct as in livedo vasculitis or Degos disease

3.8.6.3 Hyperpigmentation
The colors black, brown, blue, and gray are often included under the general term "hyperpigmentation." They can be caused by a qualitative or quantitative abnormality of the usual constituents of the skin or to the abnormal presence of a certain substance in the skin. In the latter case, the skin often displays a very unusual color, known as dyschromia.

When the predominant color is brown or black, it is mostly due to melanoderma that is an excess of melanin pigments accompanied by impairment of the epidermis or of the superficial dermis. Melanodermas are either epidermal hypermelanocytoses (increase in the number or hyperplasia of melanocytes, e.g., lentigo) or epidermal hypermelanosis (increase in the amount of epidermal melanin with no increase in the number or aspect of melanocytes, e.g., ephelides). Both mechanisms can be intricate.

If the predominant color is blue or gray, it is then a case of ceruloderma which may correspond to dermal hypermelanocytosis (abnormal presence of melanin synthesizing cells in the dermis, e.g., Ota's nevus) or to dermal hypermelaninosis (accumulation of epidermal melanin in the dermis, e.g., postinflammatory melanoderma).

3.8.6.4 Other Pigmentations
Other mechanisms are possible:
- Hyperpigmentation of hematic origin. Following an extravasation of red blood cells initially producing purpura, hemoglobin from the red blood cells are locally degraded into hemosiderin which accumulates in free form in the dermis and in macrophages, giving the skin a typical yellow, brown, or golden color, as in the most distinctive example which is venous insufficiency and to which the French refer as dermite ocre. In some cases, there is a transepidermal elimination of extravasated blood as in calcaneal petechiae (pseudochromhidrosis or black heel). Finally, intravascular thrombotic phenomena, as in angioma, are readily expressed as lesions which become black (and sometimes painful).
- Dyschromia. Pigmentation is the results of cutaneous deposit of a substance which is not usually present in the skin:
  - Exogenous pigment: the colored pigment is deposited in the skin by percutaneous absorption (tattoo, wound, etc.) or administered systemically (components or metabolites of drugs that accumulate in the skin).
  - Endogenous pigment: mostly consists in the increased blood concentration of a metabolite normally present in the body (e.g., jaundice) or a metabolic disorder with deposit of an intermediary metabolite (e.g., alkaptonuria). Apocrine chromhidrosis consists in the secretion of colored sweat. Usually of axillary location, it can also occur on the face due to ectopic apocrine glands. The coloration is caused by endogenous lipofuscins unlike "false" eccrine chromhidroses where exogenous substances or chromogenic bacteria alter sweat by coloring it.

The various mechanisms responsible for the color of macules are also applicable to other primary lesions.

On white skin particularly, the color of a lesion is an essential component of differential diagnosis. A localized modification of the skin color that is not palpable is called a macule.

Palpable and Solid Lesions

There are several types of palpable lesions that can be identified according to their content (fluid or solid), the possible presence of an alteration of the surface of the skin, and their size and location within the skin (superficial or deep).

The mechanisms underlying these lesions can be determined by the sole histopathological examination: edema, infiltration by inflammatory or tumoral cells, and substance overload (amyloidosis, mucinosis, etc.).

4.1 Papule

The papule is usually defined as a small palpable lesion, not exceeding 10 mm, with non-fluid content (Fig. 4.1). In the USA and the UK, the maximum width of a papule is restricted to 5 mm in many textbooks. Lesions are generally elevated, above the level of the adjacent skin. Seen from above, a papule may be round (Fig. 4.2), oval, umbilicated (with a small central depression) (Fig. 4.3), or polygonal. Seen in profile, it can be flat, domed, sessile, pedunculated, or acuminate

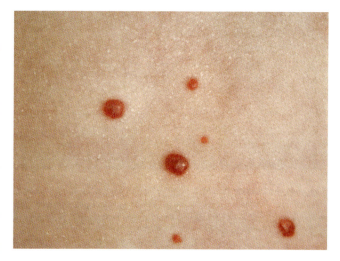

Fig. 4.2 Multiple hemispherical, dome-shaped, angiomatous papules. Diffuse neonatal hemangiomatosis. This is a potentially serious disorder because of the likelihood of visceral hemangiomas, particularly in the liver and spleen, high-output heart failure, and hypothyroidism caused by impaired secretion of a thyronine-degrading enzyme

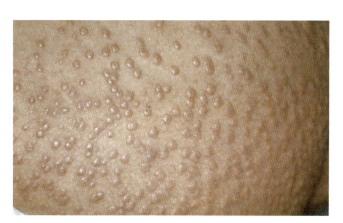

Fig. 4.1 Papules. Eruptive xanthomas. They consist of papules, i.e., palpable red or orange-yellow lesions of less than 1 cm (0.5 cm in the USA), showing no deterioration of the skin surface. They are usually numerous and of sudden onset. They are the cutaneous expression of an often major hypertriglyceridemia that can be life threatening due to the risk of pancreatitis

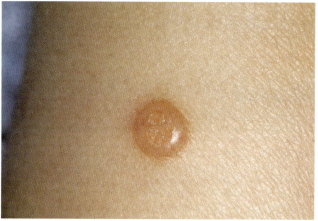

Fig. 4.3 Umbilicated papule. Molluscum contagiosum. Hemispherical pink papule, with a central depression called umbilication, highly characteristic of a virus-induced lesion. Telangiectasia may also be identified laterally. Molluscum contagiosum is a lesion related to an infection with a poxvirus. It is frequent in children. When occurring in great numbers in adults, it is essential to search for an immune deficiency

D. Lipsker, *Clinical Examination and Differential Diagnosis of Skin Lesions*, DOI 10.1007/978-2-8178-0411-8_4, © Springer-Verlag France 2013

(conical, pointed) (Fig. 4.4). The surface may be either smooth (Fig. 4.5), eroded, ulcerated, or necrotic (Fig. 4.6), covered with scales (Fig. 4.6), crusts, or scaly crusts (Fig. 4.6); hair follicles may be prominent and confer a "peau d'orange" (orange peel) appearance (Fig. 4.7). Finally the distribution pattern may or may not be follicular (Fig. 4.4).

The consistency of a papule varies depending on its nature; some lesions are very hard, others soft and depressible (Fig. 4.8). Papules that result from epidermal proliferation or deposits (e.g., plane wart, seborrheic keratosis) usually have clear-cut and rectilinear boundaries and are often rough (Fig. 4.9), whereas dermal papules

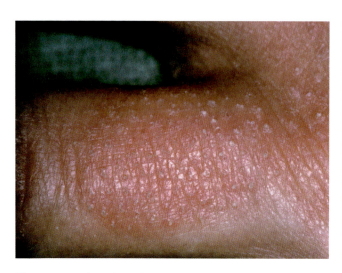

Fig. 4.4 Acuminate keratotic papules (pilar papule), on an erythematous plaque. Pityriasis rubra pilaris. These papules are cone-shaped, with a superficial apex and an epidermal base, typical of a pilar papule

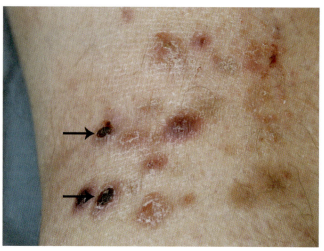

Fig. 4.6 Papules and necrotic plaques. Lymphomatoid papulosis. These papules and red plaques become scaly, crusty, and necrotic (*arrows*). They are covered with hemorrhagic crust. This is a typical progression of lymphomatoid papulosis, an auto-abortive lymphoma conferring an increased risk of Hodgkin's disease, anaplastic lymphoma, and mycosis fungoides

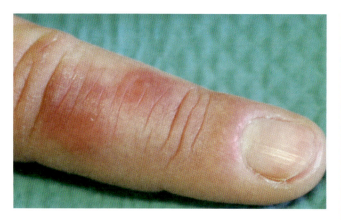

Fig. 4.5 Red, smooth, edematous papules, without alteration of the skin surface. Chilblain (pernio). These papules are poorly defined and erythematous. Chilblain is characterized by its location on extremities and its onset in cold and humid conditions. It is mostly idiopathic and can also reveal disorders such as myelomonocytic leukemia, lupus erythematosus, antiphospholipid antibody syndrome, cryopathy, or Aicardi-Goutieres syndrome in infants

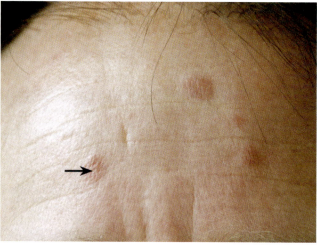

Fig. 4.7 Erythematous papules. Lever's granuloma. Note the protruding hair follicles conferring a "peau d'orange" (*orange peel*) appearance (*arrow*) characteristic of this disorder, mostly located on the face

(e.g., granuloma annulare) are smoother and borders are less defined (Fig. 4.10). Papules must be distinguished from other palpable lesions which can be larger (plaques, nodules, tumors), fluid-filled (vesicles, bullae), or mainly due to alteration of the lesion's surface (cutaneous horn, keratosis), which are also called keratotic papules.

The term *tuber* should not be used. It is a palpable intradermal lesion, either flat or barely elevated. Therefore, it is merely an intradermal papule (Fig. 4.11). These lesions often become chronic or tend to leave a scar on regression (e.g., lupus vulgaris). They are circumscribed and movable, relatively to the hypodermis.

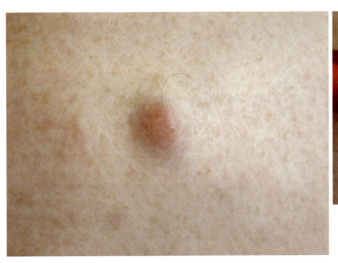
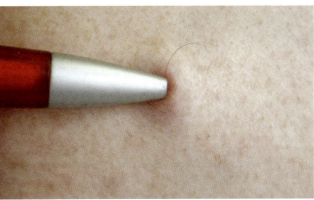

Fig. 4.8 Depressible exophytic papule. Neurofibroma. A papule is rarely depressible. It is particularly found in neurofibroma, anetoderma, certain nevi, piezogenic papules, and pendulum

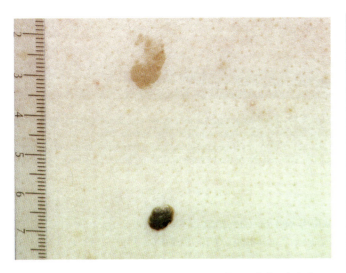
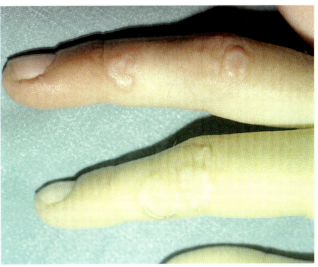

Fig. 4.9 *Dark brown* papule and *light brown* plaque. Seborrheic keratoses. Note the highly rectilinear boundaries; these two lesions seem "laid" on the skin. This is characteristic of epidermal papules. Compare the borders with those of the lesion on Fig. 4.10. Seborrheic keratosis is the result of proliferation of keratinocytes, the cells of the epidermis. It is a benign and very common lesion, especially in patients over 60 years old

Fig. 4.10 Papules and plaques in annular configuration. Granuloma annulare. Note the borders of this lesion: they are less rectilinear and less clear-cut than those of Fig. 4.9. The skin appears lifted by an underlying lesion. This semiological aspect characterizes dermal lesions; i.e., at the microscopic level, granuloma annulare is a granulomatous inflammation of the dermis ("palisading granuloma")

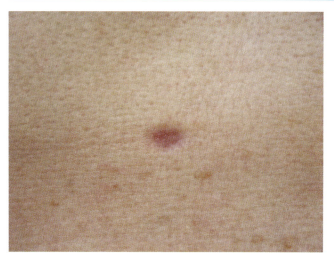

Fig. 4.11 Intradermal papule. Fibroma. The lesion has a very firm consistency on palpation. This papule is depressed below the skin surface. Pinching between thumb and forefinger forms small cavities which partially cover the lesion (*dimple sign*). This sign is characteristic of fibroma

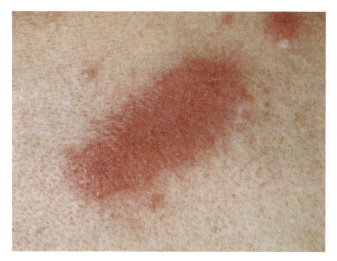

Fig. 4.12 Plaque. Sweet syndrome. Plaque is a palpable lesion measuring more than 1 cm, horizontally spread (superficially) rather than vertically (in height or depth). In this example, this is a red plaque with unaltered surface (except for a discrete scaly central area). Sweet syndrome is a neutrophilic disease (see Chap. 15); diagnosis is based on skin biopsy. Skin lesions are often associated with fever and joint pain. Sweet syndrome may reveal a blood disorder, an infection, an autoinflammatory disease, or a connective tissue disease, which must all be investigated

4.2   Plaque

The term plaque refers to raised lesions, wider than 1 cm (0.5 cm in the USA) more superficially spread than vertically raised (e.g., Sweet syndrome, Fig. 4.12). Some plaques are formed by the confluence of papules, while others are lesions measuring straightaway more than 1 cm. The various semiological aspects discussed for papules also apply to plaques,

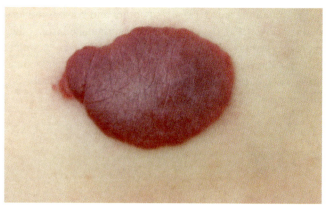

Fig. 4.13 Wine-colored, angiomatous red plaque. Hemangioma. Smooth lesion displaying the characteristic color of angiomatous lesions. Hemangioma is a tumor appearing in the postnatal period in nearly 10 % of infants. The progression includes a growth phase followed by involution and ending up with scarring between the ages of 5 and 8

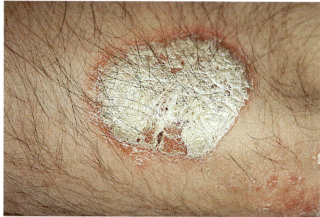

Fig. 4.14 Erythematosquamous plaque. Psoriasis. Lesion measuring more than 1 cm, more superficially spread than vertically raised (plaque). The skin surface is altered and forms white scales that can be easily removed. Note the clear delimitation, characteristic of psoriasis

which can be angiomatous (e.g., hemangioma, Fig. 4.13), scaly erythematous (e.g., psoriasis, Fig. 4.14), and erosive (e.g., extramammary Paget's disease, Fig. 4.15).

Lichenification is thickening of the skin with exaggeration of its creases, where normal skin markings become visible (Fig. 4.16). More or less prominent papules develop within these defined markings. A yellowish brown or deep purple pigmentation is often observed, as well as small adherent scales and excoriations. It is actually an intricate lesion which had historically been listed among papules and plaques in French treaties, whereas it is more a matter of nosology than semiology. It is the consequence of pruritus complicated by repeated scratching.

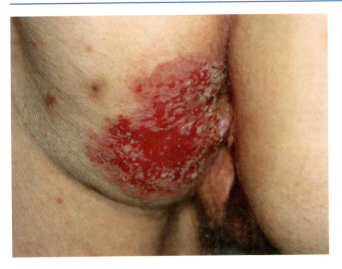

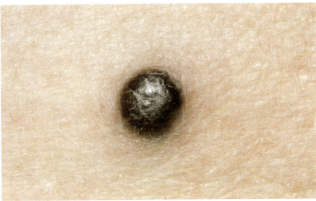

Fig. 4.17 Nodule. Melanoma metastasis. A nodule is a palpable lesion of more than 1 cm, spread vertically (in height or depth) rather than horizontally (superficially). Any hardened nodule is suspected to be a metastasis

Fig. 4.15 Erosive and macerated plaque. Extramammary Paget's disease. The presence in the inguinopelvic area of an erosive leukokeratotic plaque and/or macerated white plaques is always suspected of being an extramammary Paget's disease. This disease is an apocrine cancer with good prognosis, although it is a marker of an associated regional neoplasia in approximately 15 % of cases

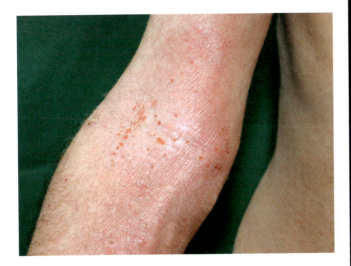

Fig. 4.16 Erythematous plaque with accentuation of the cutaneous microrelief. Lichenification. It is the consequence of scratching or repeated friction. Also note the linear excoriations

4.3 Nodule and Related Lesions

The nodule is a non-fluid-filled palpable mass, of more than 10 mm (5 mm in the USA) (Fig. 4.17). Nodule usually means a round or hemispherical lesion. Some authors call *tumor* any nodule of more than 20 mm (Fig. 4.18). Generally tumors are not inflammatory and tend to grow.

Nodules are usually located on the dermis and/or hypodermis. Nodules as well as tumors may contain surface alterations such as ulceration (e.g., squamous cell carcinoma, Fig. 4.19) and be polylobed (e.g., apocrine carcinoma, Fig. 4.20).

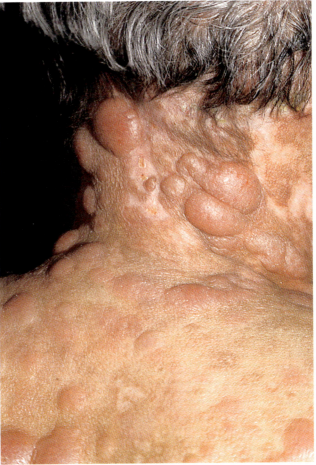

Fig. 4.18 Multiple nodules and tumors. Mycosis fungoides. Several tumor lesions on skin with dyschromia including both hypopigmented and hyperpigmented areas. Mycosis fungoides is usually an indolent T-cell lymphoma occurring as macules (cf. Fig. 18.2). Less than 20 % of patients will evolve to these potentially lethal types of tumor

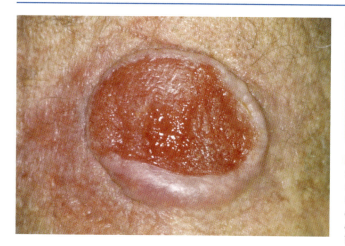

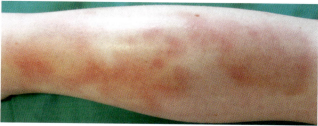

Fig. 4.21 Deep-seated inflammatory nodules ("nouures" in the French terminology). Erythema nodosum. Nodules that extend deeply subcutaneously, often slightly or barely elevated, and inflammatory (red, sensitive, and warm) are typical for erythema nodosum. Also note the coloration of these lesions which evolves as that of a bruise, through different colors: red, purple, blue, green, yellow, and brown. This bruise-like color evolution is typical of erythema nodosum

Fig. 4.19 Ulcerated nodule (tumor). Squamous cell carcinoma. The steady growth of a nodule and its ulceration are the two signs enabling to suspect the malignant nature of this lesion

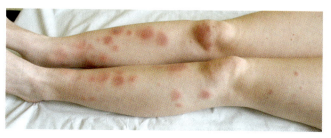

Fig. 4.22 Plaques and deep-seated nodules. Erythema nodosum. Red papules and plaques on the legs and thighs. Palpation allows assessing their depth. Between thumb and forefinger bent in hook, it is indeed possible to clearly feel the deep extent which goes beyond the elevated visible part of the lesion, indicating subcutaneous involvement. The skin cannot be folded on the lesions, showing a dermal involvement

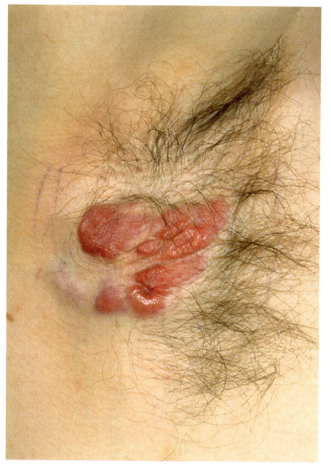

Fig. 4.20 Multilobular nodule (tumor). Axillary apocrine carcinoma. Note the multilobular nature of this cancer of the axillary apocrine glands. The multilobed feature is common in another malignant skin tumor: dermatofibrosarcoma protuberans

Normal skin is movable on the hypodermis. If the skin can be slid over the nodule, then the nodule is located in the hypodermis. However, if it seems attached to the skin surface (i.e., if it moves together with the skin, as a whole), then it is dermal or dermo-hypodermal. Any large nodule (often of more than 5 cm) extended into the hypodermis is called a *nouure* in the French terminology, the hallmark of erythema nodosum (Figs. 4.21 and 4.22). There is no equivalent designation in the English dermatologic terminology and those lesions should be referred to as inflammatory deep-seated nodules. Only deep palpation allows detecting these lesions in their early phase. Strong enough pressure must be exerted and the subcutaneous induration must be grabbed quite deeply between thumb and fingers, bent in hooks, to be able to assess its characteristics: dimension, consistency, sensitivity, etc. *Gums* (gumma) are produced subcutaneously and appear as deep-seated nodules during their crude phase (Fig. 4.23a). These nodules then enter a softening stage, which starts at the center of the gum (Fig. 4.23b) and ends with ulceration accompanied by weeping of a particular type of fluid (e.g., syphilitic gumma).

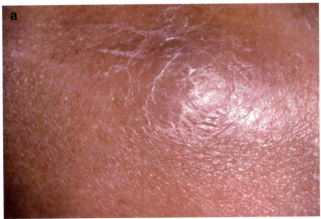

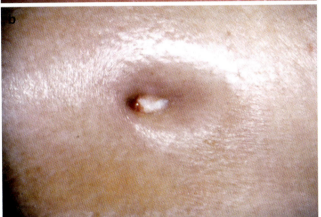

Fig. 4.23 Gum. Syphilis. Nodule (**a**) evolving to softening of its center and ulceration (**b**), with weeping of a liquid described as gummy

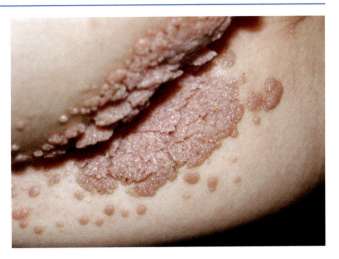

Fig. 4.24 Vegetations. Condyloma. Multiple lesions, filiform excrescences conferring a digitated or lobulated appearance in a "cockscomb" shape. Also note the smaller lesions which are papules; however, close inspection shows a tendency to lobulation

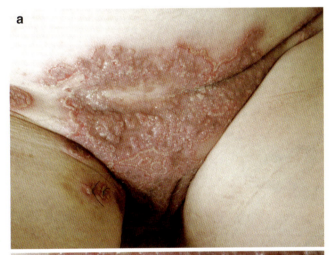

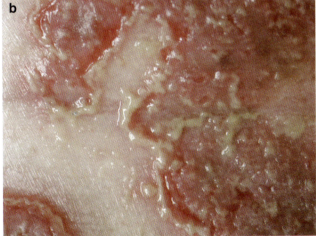

4.4 Vegetations and Verrucosis

Vegetations are filiform, digitated, or lobulated excrescences, branched in a cauliflower-like pattern and of soft consistency (e.g., venereal vegetations, Fig. 4.24). The surface of the lesion is formed by a thinned, pink-colored epidermis or covered with weeping erosions and ulcerations (e.g., venereal vegetation, iododerma). Traumatized lesions bleed easily. So-called vegetating lesions form erythematous-erosive plaques covered with small papules and/or lobulated pustules (Fig. 4.25). These are demarcated by numerous confluent pustules, aligned in a characteristic serpiginous track. Strictly speaking, these are not solid palpable lesions; they are mentioned here precisely to avoid confusion with vegetations. *Verrucosis* are filiform, digitated, or lobulated excrescences, sometimes branched in a cauliflower-like pattern and covered with an often grayish and more or less thick, callous, and keratotic coating (Fig. 4.26) (e.g., wart, seborrheic keratosis).

Fig. 4.25 Vegetating lesions. Pemphigoid. Large erosive zone (**a**) with confluent pustules in a serpiginous pattern (**b**), characteristic of so-called vegetating lesions. Vegetating lesions are mentioned here to avoid confusion with vegetations (Fig. 4.24), since they are not solid palpable lesions. These vegetating lesions are particularly often seen in inflammatory bowel disease (*CIBD* chronic inflammatory bowel disease). However, they also occur in autoimmune bullous dermatoses (pemphigus vegetans, bullous pemphigoid)

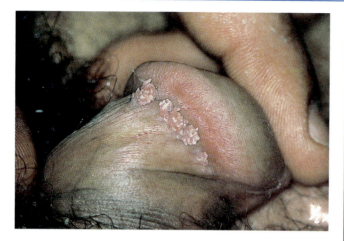

Fig. 4.26 Verrucosis. Condyloma. Lesions resemble vegetations seen on Fig. 4.24, i.e., filiform excrescences, although their surface is covered with a firm, yellow, keratotic coating. These lesions are called verrucosis

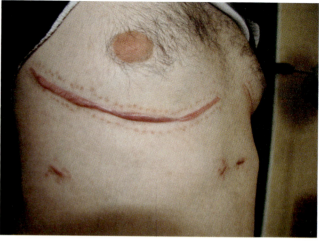

Fig. 4.28 Cord. Hypertrophic scar (lung transplant). This is a linear lesion resembling a cord. A scar may initially be hypertrophic and then spontaneously flatten. As opposed to keloids (cf. Fig. 12.60), hypertrophic scars do not have lateral extensions in a crab-leg pattern

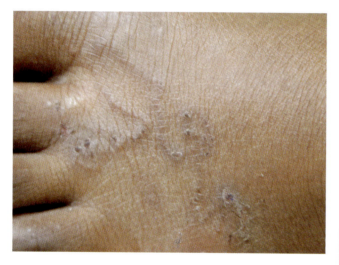

Fig. 4.27 Serpiginous cord. Larva migrans. This lesion is pruritic and barely movable ("creeping dermatitis"). It is the result of intradermal migration of a larva (usually *Ancylostoma caninum*). Also note excoriations and frequent crusts resulting from scratching. This lesion stands between a furrow and a cord (it is indeed an intradermal tunnel made by a parasite). However, the term furrow usually describes lesions of less than 1 mm, where the parasite is located in the epidermis; here, it is located in the dermis

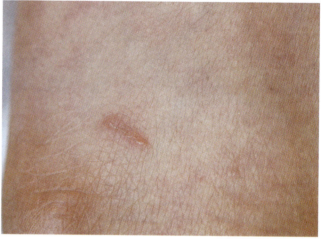

Fig. 4.29 Furrow. Scabies. This is a sinuous lesion measuring only a few millimeters, on a red background. It is typical of a scabies furrow, thus confirming the diagnosis of scabies in a patient with scratching. These lesions must be carefully searched, especially on the fingers, the palms, and the wrists

4.5 Other Palpable Lesions

A linear *cord* is a more easily palpable than visible lesion and offers the feeling of a cord or a string, on palpation. These lesions are linear and more or less sinuous (Fig. 4.27). Their size is highly variable. They are listed as primary lesions since they are easily identified. They include various lesions such as the palpable cords of hypertrophic scars (Fig. 4.28), superficial venous thromboses (cf. Fig. 15.3), temporal arteritis (or Horton's disease), or the palpable cord of an interstitial granulomatous dermatitis.

A *furrow* is a small tunnel inside the skin which usually contains a parasite (e.g., scabies, Fig. 4.29); this lesion is often millimeter wide and hardly visible and/or palpable.

4.6 Clinicopathological Correlations: Mechanisms

A lesion may become palpable for the following reasons.

4.6.1 Anomaly Is Located in the Epidermis

These lesions have sharp, rectilinear borders. They appear as laid on the skin and can thus be distinguished from dermal papules:

- Epidermis is thickened and there is ortho- and parakeratotic hyperkeratosis: it is then a rough lesion, characteristic of keratosis. Other epidermal and/or dermal lesions may be associated.
- Epidermis harbors a tunnel dug by a parasite, which becomes a furrow.

4.6.2 Anomaly Is Located in the Dermis

It may be:

- An excess or modification of one of the normal components of the dermis, such as collagen bundles or elastic fibers. In the case of excess collagen (e.g., collagen hamartoma or collagenoma), the resulting lesion consists of papules and/or homogeneous plaques, without alteration of the skin surface and of normal skin color. Unlike epidermal papules, they have a round border because they elevate the epidermis. Lesions are more firm in the case of sclerosis, which is a thickening and densification of collagen bundles.
- The presence in the dermis of an otherwise absent substance: amyloid material, mucin, lipoprotein, etc. Lesions are generally more firm, although clinical characteristics are close to those of papules and plaques formed by excessive collagen bundles.
- An infiltration of inflammatory cells with variable topography (superficial and/or deep perivascular, interstitial, diffuse, etc.). These lesions are almost always erythematous, since the perivascular infiltrate causes vasodilation.
- Tumoral proliferation of cells normally located in the dermis (e.g., dermatofibrosarcoma) or of cells of other origin (e.g., metastases). These lesions are often indurated. They have a tendency to grow and usually evolve into nodules and tumors. Ulceration is common.
- Significant edema of the dermis: it then consists of papules and plaques which are not very firm and slightly depressible. These lesions are usually transient. Urticaria is an example. In Sweet syndrome and erythema multiforme, the simultaneous presence of significant edema and cell infiltrate explains the firmness of the lesions compared to simple urticaria lesions.

4.6.3 Anomaly Is Located Deeper in the Hypodermis or the Adjacent Structures

Any deep lesion may elevate the dermis and epidermis. In some cases, the skin may not be raised but a firm lesion can be felt on deep palpation between thumb and forefinger bent in hooks. Deep involvement produces infiltrated plaques or nodules. The bruise-like color evolution characterizes erythema nodosum.

Lesions can be the result of:

- Cell infiltration (inflammatory or tumoral) or sclerosis of the inter-adipose septa. Inflammation of the inter-adipose septa characterizes erythema nodosum.
- Infiltration (inflammatory or tumoral) of adipose lobules, consisting in panniculitis.
- Thrombosis or inflammation of hypodermal vessels, producing linear, layered lesions, sometimes associated with livedo when blood vessels lined with muscle tissue are affected.
- Deeper involvement underneath the hypodermis, requiring deep and large biopsy (at least 1 cm) in order to establish proper diagnosis. In this case, the skin can be folded over the lesion.

The color of the various palpable lesions is determined using the same mechanisms as those underlying the color of macules (cf. Chap. 3).

Palpable lesions may be fluid-filled or solid. Elevated solid lesions are separated according to the presence of a possible alteration of the skin surface, to their size, and to their depth. A papule is a palpable lesion of less than 1 cm; a plaque is a palpable lesion of more than 1 cm, superficially spread rather than vertically raised. A nodule is a lesion of more than 1 cm, spread in all three dimensions, and is often hemispherical or spherical.

Fluid-Filled Lesions

5.1 Vesicle

Vesicles are lesions of less than 5 mm that contain (clear) fluid (Fig. 5.1). In order to distinguish vesicles from small papules of solid content, it is sometimes necessary to puncture the top of a vesicle by means of a vaccinostyle (a pointed lancet) or a small needle, to make sure it is fluid-filled. Vesicles are sometimes conspicuous and produce a translucent lesion, which can be round (hemispherical), conical (acuminate), or depressed (umbilicate) (see Fig. 2.11). However, they are often fragile and temporary and can burst

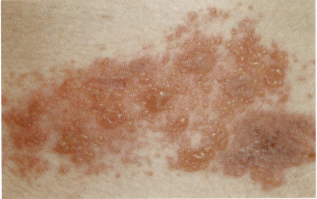

Fig. 5.2 Vesicles. Zoster. Grouped vesicles on an erythematous background. Several elements are characteristic of the viral nature of the vesicles on one side and of its cause, zoster, on the other. The gray color and the umbilication are typical of the viral nature. Clustering is typical of herpetic infections. The metameric arrangement immediately indicates zoster (shingles). Unlike vesicles of dermatitis (eczema), these lesions do not evolve towards weeping but may evolve into a painful cutaneous necrosis

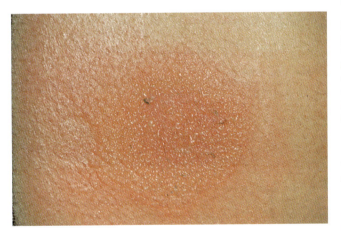

Fig. 5.1 Vesicles. Acute dermatitis (eczema). Multiple confluent and translucent vesicles on an erythematous background, as observed in acute allergic contact dermatitis. A vesicle is a fluid-filled lesion of less than 5 mm. It is one of the primary lesions of dermatitis. The usual course of dermatitis includes erythema, vesicles, weeping erosion, crusting, and recovery. Intense pruritus is present at all stages. The absence of pruritus requires that the diagnosis be revised. The vesicle observed in dermatitis is the prototype example of vesicles that develop weeping, which reflects the pathogenic mechanism of spongiosis. Spongiosis indicates intercellular epidermal edema. Viral vesicles produced by other mechanisms (necrosis) do not evolve towards weeping

and produce weeping, erosions, and crusting, borders of crusts being rounded, fragmented, or polycyclic. Microscopic vesicles may produce clinical aspects appearing as erythematosquamous or papular. Vesicles evolving towards weeping usually indicate a spongiosis from the histopathological point of view; they are typical of eczema ("dermatitis"). Conversely, vesicles evolving towards umbilication and/or necrosis without weeping often reflect a viral cytopathogenic effect, as in infections caused by herpesvirus or zoster/varicella virus (Fig. 5.2). Oblong vesicles found on extremities are characteristic of hand-foot-and-mouth syndrome (Fig. 5.3). A vesicle should not be mistaken with a hidrocystoma (Fig. 5.4), a translucent sudoral cyst, or pseudovesicles of lymphedema (Fig. 5.5).

D. Lipsker, *Clinical Examination and Differential Diagnosis of Skin Lesions*, DOI 10.1007/978-2-8178-0411-8_5, © Springer-Verlag France 2013

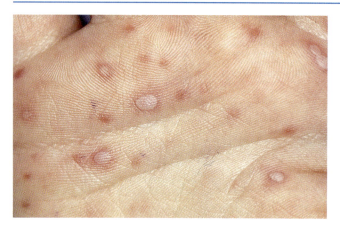

Fig. 5.3 Oblong vesicles. Hand-foot-and-mouth disease. The *gray color* is characteristic of a viral lesion. Note the oblong shape and the erythematous border of these lesions. In this disorder, the lesions are located on the palms and soles. The disorder itself is caused by a Coxsackie virus infection (benign form) or an echovirus (more serious form due to neuromeningeal and cardiopulmonary risks). Buccal vesicular erosive involvement may also exist

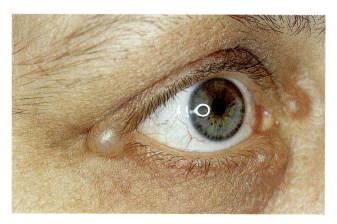

Fig. 5.4 Differential diagnosis of a vesicle. Telangiectatic translucent papule. Hidrocystoma. This is a thin-wall sudoriparous cyst located in the superficial dermis. This cyst may resemble a vesicle and can be emptied through puncturing. Its fluid is however more viscous. It is almost always located around the eyes

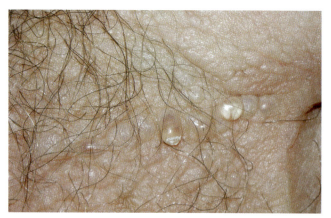

Fig. 5.5 Differential diagnosis of a vesicle. Pseudovesicles of lymphedema. Penoscrotal lymphedema. In the course of lymphedema where lymph accumulates in the cutaneous collectors, the appearance may be that of a vesicle or a bulla. Note also the numerous skin-colored papules of lymphedema. These papules can be completely flattened by applying prolonged finger pressure

5.2 Bulla

Bullae are lesions of more than 5 mm containing (clear) fluid (Fig. 5.6). Subepidermal bullae have a solid roof and lie on normal, erythematous, or urticarial skin (e.g., pemphigoid, Fig. 5.7, or porphyria cutanea tarda, Fig. 5.6). They are distinguished from epidermal bullae, which are fragile and rupture spontaneously, thus appearing as a collarette-bordered erosion (e.g., pemphigus, Fig. 5.8). Bullae may contain clear (Fig. 5.6), cloudy (Fig. 5.9), or hemorrhagic (Fig. 5.10; see Fig. 28.2) fluid. In the case of a very superficial bullous lesion, located beneath the stratum corneum, its extreme fragility explains its post-bullous presentation, i.e., usually round scaly crusts (e.g., bullous impetigo; see Figs. 2.8 and 5.15).

The clear fluid contents of vesicles and bullae tend to gradually become cloudy if the vesicles do not rupture. Therefore, it is the initial color of the fluid which determines the nature of the lesions.

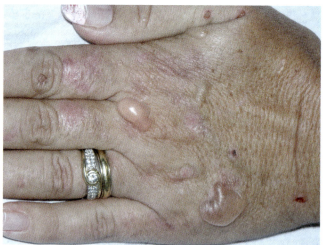

Fig. 5.6 Tense bullae. Porphyria cutanea tarda. Note also the red, shiny, and mildly depressed scars and visible crusted erosion on the thumb root. The simultaneous presence of both these lesions on the back and the hands is highly suggestive of the diagnosis of porphyria cutanea tarda, a photo-triggered disorder

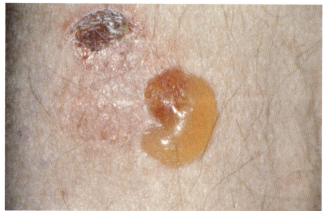

Fig. 5.7 Bulla. Crust. Pemphigoid. Tense bulla and, above, crust that appeared on a post-bullous erosion

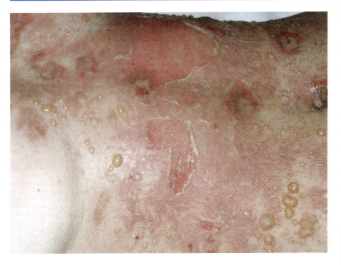

Fig. 5.8 Erosion, erythema, bullae. Pemphigus. Those affected by pemphigus have a marked mucocutaneous fragility, which explains the numerous erosions following rupture of the bullae and positive Nikolsky's sign (refer to Fig. 8.3)

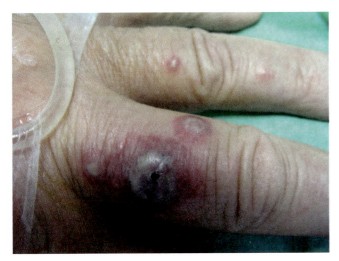

Fig. 5.9 Pustule and purulent bulla on a purpuric background. Cutaneous reaction to azathioprine. Onset of pustules on a purpuric background is rare and should always first and foremost suggest a septicemia (particularly due to gonococci, when the lesions are periarticular, and to meningococci) and/or an endocarditis. This patient has Crohn's disease which predisposes to pustular reactions

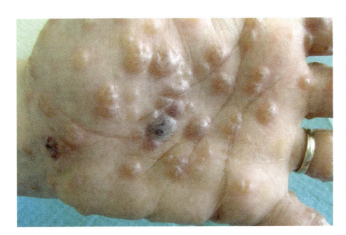

Fig. 5.10 Confluent multilocular vesicle and bullae. Dyshidrosis. These are tense, multilocular, and highly pruritic vesicles. Note certain hemorrhagic lesions

5.3 Pustule

When fluid contained in the lesion is primarily cloudy or purulent, it is a pustule (Fig. 5.11). Pustules are less than 5 mm in diameter; a purulent lesion measuring more than 5 mm is called a purulent bulla (Fig. 5.12). Among pustules, follicular lesions which are acuminate and centered on hair follicles (e.g., folliculitis, Fig. 5.13) are distinguished from non-follicular lesions, which are generally more planar, not acuminate, and whitish (Fig. 5.14). The second type of pustule is generally located in the epidermis under the stratum

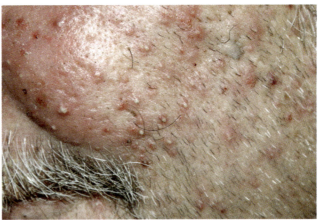

Fig. 5.11 Pustules. Cutaneous drug reaction to EGFR (epidermal growth factor receptor) inhibitors. The pustule is a fluid-filled lesion of at least 5 mm diameter. Its fluid content is primarily purulent. Also note the presence of red papules and papulopustules (pustules occurring on a raised red lesion); some pustules are centered on hair follicles and correspond to folliculitis. Note the absence of comedones (blackhead), which are always present in acne. Such pustular reactions commonly occur with drugs that inhibit tyrosine kinases

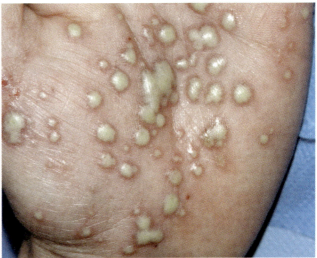

Fig. 5.12 Pustules and palmar purulent bullae. Crohn's disease. Note that even the very initial, small-sized lesions are immediately pustular. Therefore, they are not secondarily infected lesions. Compare with Fig. 5.10 (dyshidrosis). Pustular eruptions can be seen in most autoinflammatory diseases, such as Crohn's disease

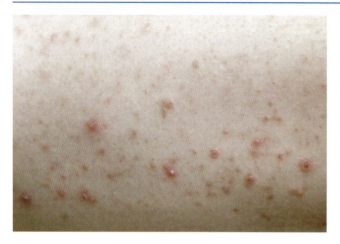

Fig. 5.13 Follicular pustules. Folliculitis. When a pustule is centered on a hair follicle, it is known as folliculitis. The hair or vellus cannot always be seen; however, the pointed shape (acuminate) of these pustules is characteristic. Also note the macules and pustules rimmed by a scaling collarette, typical of post-pustular lesions

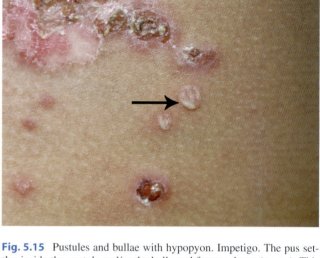

Fig. 5.15 Pustules and bullae with hypopyon. Impetigo. The pus settles inside the pustule and/or the bulla and forms a layer (*arrow*). This phenomenon is called hypopyon. It is typical of stratum corneum pustules. Also note the honey-colored crusts typical of impetigo

5.4 Clinicopathological Correlations: Mechanisms

Fluid-filled lesions can be intraepidermal or dermal. The higher they are located the more fragile they are, as they can rupture easily. The lesions situated in the upper stratum corneum are hence transient and, after rupturing, leave a round area bordered by a collarette.

A lesion may become filled with fluid for the following reasons:

- An intraepidermal and intercellular edema (named spongiosis) separates the keratinocytes and may lead to a vesicle or an intraepidermal bulla. These lesions evolve towards weeping and are pruritic.
- Necrosis of the keratinocytes can also lead to formation of vesicles and bullae. It may be a reticular necrosis of keratinocytes, resulting into an umbilicated vesicle which evolves into non-weeping necrosis, particularly in herpesvirus infections. These vesicles can also be pruritic. Keratinocyte necrosis can also be diffuse and therefore lead to formation of vesicles and bullae, followed by a more or less extensive epidermolysis with crusting, in disorders such as certain serious cutaneous drug reactions, lichen, or lupus erythematosus.

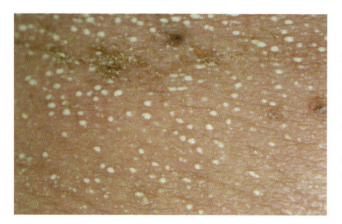

Fig. 5.14 Pustules. Pustular allergic contact dermatitis (caused by ketoprofen). Allergic contact dermatitis is usually vesicular. It can rarely be pustular. Also note the presence of some yellow, honey-colored crusts as well as the milky color of the pustules

corneum and is very superficial, sometimes showing only circular micro-erosions. The collection sometimes settles within the pustular material, forming a layer or hypopyon (e.g., subcorneal pustular dermatosis of Sneddon and Wilkinson or impetigo, Fig. 5.15).

- A vesicle or a bulla can also result from the separation of keratinocytes due to failure of the inter-keratinocyte adhesion mechanisms, thus producing a cleavage picture known as acantholytic, where floating acantholytic keratinocytes can be observed. This phenomena can be seen in autoantibody-mediated disorders, where antibodies target adhesion proteins of epidermal cells (pemphigus), or in genetic diseases where these mechanisms do not function properly (Darier's disease, Hailey-Hailey disease, and other rare inherited diseases where the intraepidermal adhesion systems are altered).

- The entire epidermis – of normal aspect – can be raised by a vesicle or a bulla in the following circumstances:
  - By a more or less inflammatory edema of the dermis, underlain by numerous mechanisms
  - By poor anchoring of the epidermis to the dermis, as in hereditary epidermolysis bullosa, whether junctional or dermal, where the dermo-epidermal adhesion systems are defective, and also in certain acquired autoimmune bullous dermatoses where the anchoring systems of the epidermis to the dermis are altered

- Rarely, there may exist true intradermal or dermolytic bullae, when the collagenous components are very much altered (e.g., bullous morphea) or when the dermis harbors a deposit that alters its mechanical properties (e.g., dermolytic bullae in amyloidosis).

- All major cell infiltrate that becomes located in the epidermis through a mechanism known as exocytosis may lead to a fluid-filled lesion.

If exocytosis is related to neutrophils, pustules are distinguished according to the confluence mechanism of the granular cells (unilocular or multilocular) and to their site of accumulation (stratum corneum or intraepidermal).

It is sometimes necessary to resort to puncturing with a needle, to make sure that the lesion is fluid-filled. Fluid-filled lesions of less than 5 mm are called vesicles when their fluid content is clear, and pustules when purulent. Fluid-filled lesions of more than 5 mm diameter are called bullae. The fragility of these lesions explains their transient nature and the fact that only their effects are sometimes visible: round erosions, scaling collarette, and crusts.

Some diseases cause abnormalities in the thickness and/or consistency of the skin. These need to be assessed by pinching and stretching the skin. The skin may become too hard and lose its usual suppleness or on the contrary may be too supple. These abnormalities result from pathological or physiological modifications (aging) of its connective tissue, the dermis, which is composed mostly of collagen bundles and elastic fibers.

6.1 Sclerosis

Sclerosis is an induration or hardening of the skin, which has lost its normal suppleness. The skin can no longer be pinched (Fig. 6.1b). This condition is often associated with a pigment disorder as the skin becomes hyper- and/or hypopigmented in sclerotic areas (Fig. 6.1a, b).

6.2 Skin Hyperextensibility

Skin that can abnormally be extended, but maintains normal elasticity by returning to its initial position after extension, is called hyperextensible (Fig. 6.2a). Skin hyperextensibility reflects an abnormality of the dermal collagen. It is often associated with joint hypermobility (Fig. 6.2b).

6.3 Loss of Elasticity

Alteration or loss of elastic tissue results in loss of skin elasticity. The skin subsequently becomes loose and does not recover its initial aspect after pinching; imprinted marks persist. There is spontaneous formation of wrinkles, lines, and skin folds (Fig. 6.3) and/or of an actual cutis laxa which refers to loosening of the skin which hangs and does not recover after extension (Fig. 6.4). Thus, loss of elasticity results in permanent skin folds located in areas where the skin is not usually being repeatedly folded.

6.4 Atrophy

Atrophy of the skin corresponds the reduction or loss of some or all skin components (epidermis, dermis, hypodermis, or two to three skin compartments). Epidermal or dermo-epidermal atrophy manifests as thinning of the skin and wrinkling upon superficial pinching. The skin

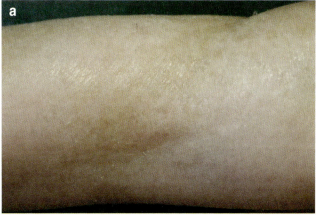

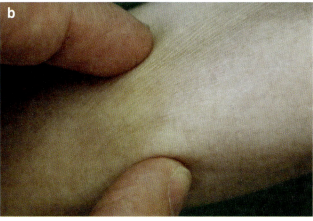

Fig. 6.1 Cutaneous sclerosis. Morphea. The skin has lost its suppleness and can no longer be folded between the thumb and index finger (**b**). Dyschromia is present, with hyper- and hypopigmented areas (**a**, **b**). Also note the skin's shiny and finely wrinkled appearance

D. Lipsker, *Clinical Examination and Differential Diagnosis of Skin Lesions*, DOI 10.1007/978-2-8178-0411-8_6, © Springer-Verlag France 2013

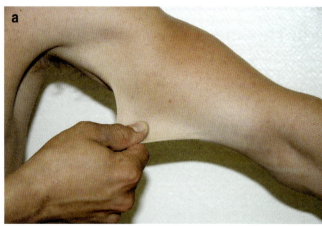
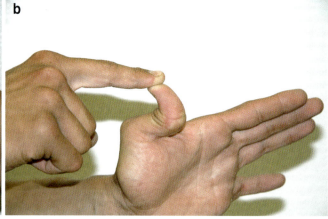

Fig. 6.2 Cutaneous (**a**) and articular (**b**) hyperextensibility. Ehlers-Danlos syndrome. The skin can be abnormally stretched but immediately returns to its initial position when released. This syndrome includes numerous genetic variants with different clinical pictures and is related to an anomaly of the connective tissue. Skin elasticity remains normal since the skin returns to its initial position when pulled. This hyperextensibility is also observed in Marfan syndrome

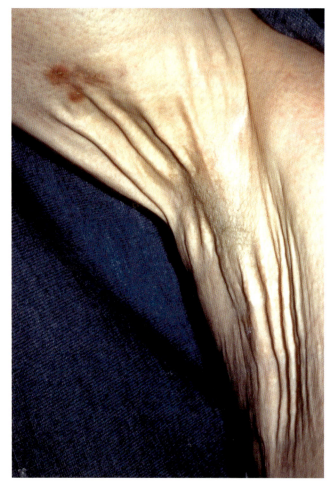

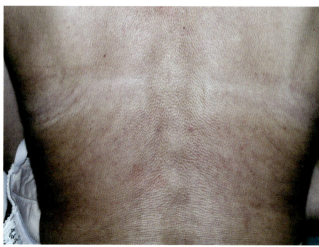

Fig. 6.4 Abnormally folded skin, skin atrophy and "peau d'orange" (*orange peel*) appearance. Cutis laxa. Cutis laxa results in loss of elasticity of the skin caused by the destruction of elastic fibers. It can be genetically determined or can be acquired as in this young woman, where it occurred secondary to cutaneous mastocytosis. Note the finely wrinkled skin in the lumbar area, as well as bigger folds on the sides. Finally, due to the complete disappearance of the elastic fiber network in the skin of this young woman, including in the peripilar adventitial dermis, hair follicles become prominent and confer this peau d'orange (*orange peel*) appearance

Fig. 6.3 Loss of elasticity. Pseudoxanthoma elasticum. Functional alteration of elastic fibers causes loss of elasticity. In this patient, it results into the formation of permanent folds in the axillae, with the appearance of "hanging skin"

loses its (micro)-relief and elasticity and takes a shiny, smooth, translucent, and pearly appearance (cf. Figs. 2.4 and 3.16). Dermal vessels become abnormally visible through the skin's transparent layers, due to thinning (Fig. 6.5).

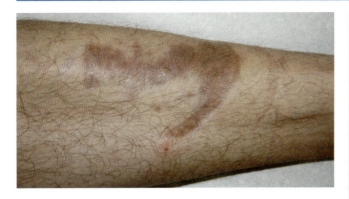

Fig. 6.5 Cutaneous atrophy. Scar. The skin is slightly depressed, pigmented, fine, shiny, and wrinkled. In some areas, it has the appearance of "cigarette paper." Also note the abnormally visible superficial skin vessels due to the extreme transparency of atrophic skin

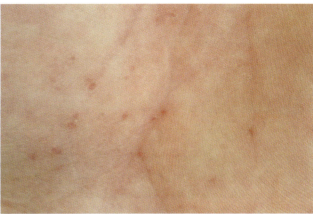

Fig. 6.7 Palmar depressions (pits). Gorlin's syndrome (basal cell nevus syndrome). This type of millimeter-wide depression on palms and soles, known as palmar pits, is almost pathognomonic of Gorlin's syndrome. This is a genetically determined disease which predisposes to the development of hundreds of basal cell carcinomas

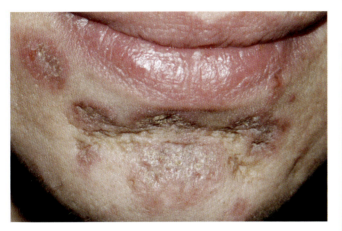

Fig. 6.6 Cutaneous depression (dermo-epidermal atrophy). Chronic lupus erythematosus (discoid type). The skin is clearly depressed, in the central part of this figure. It is thin, transparent, and slightly erythematous, both in the lower part of this figure and on the second lesion, on the left, where epidermal atrophy is predominant. Also note keratosis and the pigmentary changes with hyper- and hypopigmented areas. This type of evolution, towards highly visible and unsightly sequelae, emphasizes the seriousness of the cutaneous manifestations in this disease

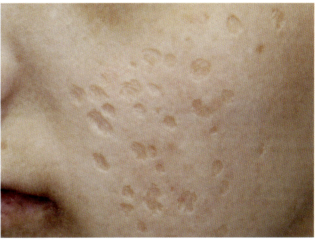

Fig. 6.8 Depressed plaque. Scars. Griscelli's syndrome. These particularly visible scars are the consequences of a chronic granulomatous inflammation which has regressed after bone marrow transplantation. This rare syndrome has several variants. This young girl had silver hair and diffuse aseptic cutaneous granulomas prior to developing macrophage activation syndrome

6.5 Cutaneous Depression

Some lesions become palpable since they produce a cutaneous depression, while the skin maintains its normal elasticity. Such depressions reflect injury of the dermis (superficial depression) and/or hypodermis (deep depression). These lesions may include an anomaly of the skin surface such as atrophy (Fig. 6.6) or thinning of the stratum corneum (hypokeratosis, Fig. 6.7). For example, a scar may produce a superficial depression and an evenly depressed plate or dell (Fig. 6.8). Stretch marks produce a very superficial linear depression (Fig. 6.9). The consequence of panniculitis (e.g., in lupus erythematosus) may manifest as a deep, cupuliform, more or less padded, or bumpy depression or gully (Fig. 6.10). These various types of depressions have not yet been described by any specific term. The term "depression" can thus be used, followed by one or more descriptive adjectives (superficial, deep, cupuliform, linear, etc.).

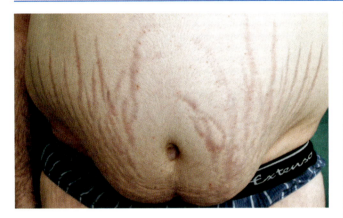

Fig. 6.9 Superficial linear depressions. Stretch marks. Stretch marks are very common and are mostly caused by rapid changes in height and weight

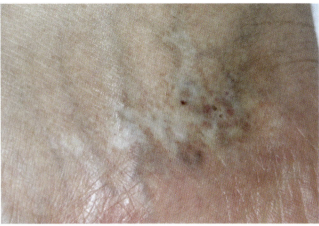

Fig. 6.11 Scleroatrophy. Atrophie blanche. This lesion is both sclerotic and atrophic. It may be caused by venous insufficiency or thrombotic microangiopathy, which can have many causes

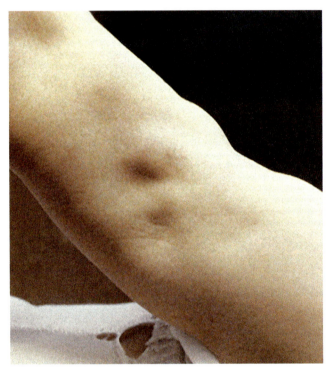

Fig. 6.10 Cupuliform depressions. Sequela of panniculitis. These depressions are caused by postinflammatory loss of hypodermal fat and have a typical cupuliform appearance ("gully")

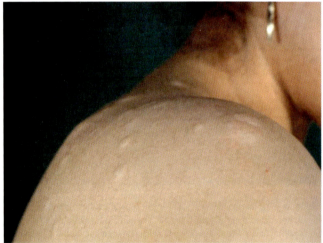

Fig. 6.12 Anetoderma. Cause was not identified. These flesh-colored lesions can be depressed. Biopsy showed complete loss of the elastic fiber network. Anetoderma appearing de novo (i.e., not on a preexisting lesion) commands a full investigation for infectious diseases (particularly HIV [human immunodeficiency virus], syphilis, and borreliosis), lymphoma, connective tissue diseases, and a thrombophilic state such as antiphospholipid antibody syndrome

6.6 Other Anomalies in Thickness and Consistency

Atrophy is often associated with cutaneous sclerosis, resulting in scleroatrophy (Fig. 6.11). Scars can thus be atrophic, scleroatrophic, or on the contrary hypertrophic. Sometimes atrophy can only be detected on palpation. Hence, palpating anetoderma is felt as penetrating an actual depression, whereas to the contrary, the skin seems to be prominent upon inspection (Fig. 6.12). Atrophoderma (vermiculatum or follicular) indicates depressed, millimeter-wide perifollicular lesions (Fig. 6.13), often associated with keratosis pilaris. These lesions may merge and produce unsightly "beehive-like" depressed plaques.

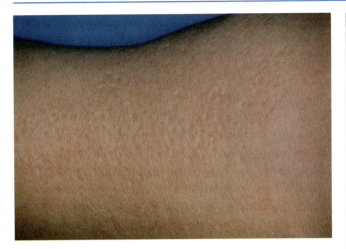

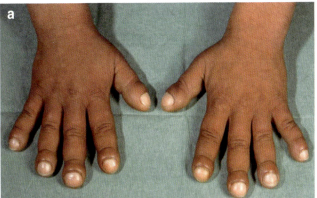

Fig. 6.13 Multiple millimeter-wide depressions. Follicular atrophoderma. Multiple, depressed, millimeter-wide lesions, of the same color as normal skin. Note the typical follicular arrangement suggested by the relatively equidistant lesions. Atrophoderma may be the sequela of a dermatosis such as acne, in which case it is often vermiculate (worm-shaped). When it seems primary in infants, it can be a skin marker for various uncommon syndromes (Bazex-Christol-Dupré, Nicolau-Balus, Rombo, Happle-Tintschert, etc.)

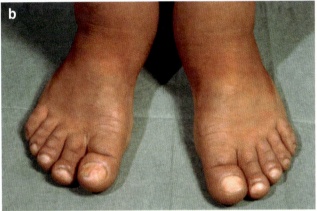

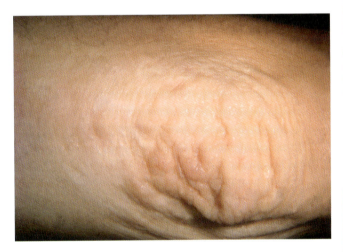

Fig. 6.15 Thickened skin on hands and feet (**a**, **b**). Pachydermoperiostosis. In this disorder, the forehead is constantly thickened and wrinkled. Periostitis is present and clubbing of the fingers is well visible on (**a**). Pachydermoperiostosis involves ruling out acromegaly and commands an investigation for cancer, since it may be paraneoplastic

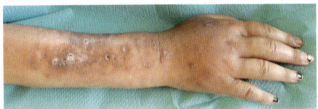

Fig. 6.14 Thick and shiny skin on the elbow. Lipoid proteinosis (Urbach-Wiethe disease, hyalinosis cutis, and mucosae). The skin is too thick, pachydermic. It is an autosomal recessive overload disorder affecting the skin, larynx (hoarseness of voice), and mouth. The overloading deposit infiltrates the tissues and causes the clinical appearance

Fig. 6.16 Thickened skin with multiple ulcerations on a background of lymphedema, particularly on the back of the hands. Puffy hand syndrome. This appearance is the consequence of subcutaneous and/or intravenous injections of substances not meant to be administered as such, particularly buprenorphine. Also note dyschromia and the pearly white sclero-cicatricial appearance

Finally, on rare occasions, the skin may become too thick (pachydermia) without being sclerotic. This can be the case in some overload disorders such as lipoid proteinosis (hyalinosis cutis and mucosae of Urbach-Wiethe) (Fig. 6.14), due to abnormal dermal deposits. It is also the case in pachydermoperiostosis, where there is hypertrophia of tissues composing the skin and distal bones (Fig. 6.15). Lastly, chronic lymphedema may cause thickening of the skin, which occurs, for example, in puffy hand syndrome (Fig. 6.16). This syndrome is related to repeated subcutaneous and/or intravenous injections of substances not meant to be administered as such, particularly buprenorphine.

6.7   Clinicopathological Correlations: Mechanisms

Upon microscopic examination, alterations of the elastic tissue may be reflected by:

- Elastolysis, i.e., decline of elastic fibers, which become fine and fragmented and finally disappear completely. Orcein staining is sometimes necessary in order to reveal this rarefaction. The skin retains the imprinted fold. When elastolysis affects the superficial and/or middle dermis, the skin becomes thin and wrinkled, usually containing a prominence appearing as perifollicular anetoderma. When mainly located in the superficial dermis, lesions can be millimeter-wide white papules.
- Elastorrhexis, where the elastic fibers of the reticular dermis are thickened, curled up, and chopped. In pseudoxanthoma elasticum, the elastic fibers calcify. Accumulation of calcified elastic fibers explains the formation of palpable yellow lesions. However, in "papular elastorrhexis," the elastic fibers tend to disappear while collagen bundles are thickened and homogenized and there is an excess of fibrocytes. The clinical appearance is therefore closer to palpable lesions, due to excess collagen (collagenoma).
- Elastoderma, where there is abnormal accumulation of pleomorphic and noncalcified elastic fibers. Finally, elastic fibers are thickened in elastomas; in Buschke-Ollendorff syndrome, they are thickened and intermingled; in actinic elastosis, they thicken and form amorphous aggregates. Most of these lesions have a variable yellow coloration.

Collagen alterations may correspond to:

- Sclerosis, which is a densification and thickening of collagen bundles causing indurated skin that cannot be folded, as in morphea and scleroderma.
- Hyalinization of collagen bundles, mostly in the superficial dermis, resulting in a white pearly skin, barely stretchable, as in lichen sclerosus.
- Rarefaction of collagen bundles during dermal atrophy (see below).
- Functional alteration of collagen, as in Ehlers-Danlos syndromes. Usually it is not reflected morphologically at the microscopic level, while there is a marked cutaneous hyperlaxity.

Some sclerodermiform conditions are identified by other microscopic anomalies:

- Amyloid infiltration (amyloidosis) or mucin infiltration (scleromyxedema) of the dermis
- Sclerotic or sclero-mucinous infiltration rich in fibrocytes (nephrogenic systemic fibrosis) or eosinophils (eosinophilic fasciitis or Shulman's syndrome)

Histopathologically, cutaneous atrophy is caused by various mechanisms resulting in loss of substance. This loss of substance may affect the thickness of the epidermis, which becomes atrophic through flattening, reduction of the number of cell layers, and disappearance of the rete ridges. This gives unusual thinness and transparency to the skin, especially when there is an associated dermal atrophy. Sometimes, circumscribed hypokeratosis may produce a round depression in areas where the stratum corneum is thickened (palms and soles). This depression is exclusively related to a reduced thickness of the stratum corneum. When the dermis is affected, its thickness is diminished by a decrease in collagen bundles and their fragmentation or rarefaction. Sclerosis may also cause cutaneous depression by densification and shrinkage of collagen bundles. Finally, spontaneous or postinflammatory disappearance of all or part of hypodermal fat (lipoatrophy) produces a cupuliform depression (gully). All these anomalies can be isolated or associated with each other.

Palpation and pinching of the skin enable to identify these lesions.

Schematically, loss of cutaneous suppleness indicates a sclerosis; hyperextensibility indicates a collagen alteration; and extremely loose skin that retains the imprinted fold indicates an alteration of elastic tissue. An overly thin, wrinkled, transparent, and/or depressed skin is atrophic. A cupuliform depression is almost always the sign of the disappearance of adipose lobules in the hypodermis.

All lesions described so far may also include an alteration of the surface of the skin and thus produce intricate lesions (e.g., a papule may become necrotic = necrotic papule). Some lesions known as "primary," with an initially normal surface, will evolve towards an alteration of the skin surface. This observation explains the historical designation of "secondary lesions" for skin surface alterations. However, it is an inaccurate term since these lesions can be initially present in numerous conditions and are not necessarily an evolution of a "primary lesion." For teaching purposes, these lesions have already been defined and briefly covered in Chap. 2. A more comprehensive description is presented here, although readers may also refer to the illustrations in Chap. 2.

Normal skin is smooth and dry (except for sweat), and the microrelief is apparent. Soft scratching using a Brocq's curette (or otherwise rubbing with the finger or a black piece of cloth) does not cause scale removal.

The standard terminology for these alterations of the skin surface is as follows.

7.1 Skin Surface Is Too Thin

The skin becomes transparent and wrinkled. This anomaly is called *atrophy* (cf. Figs. 2.4 and 3.16 and also cf. Chap. 6). When affecting mainly the epidermis, atrophy is in fact more visible than palpable.

7.2 Skin Surface Is Thickened

The skin then becomes yellow, hard, and rough.

Keratosis is defined as a thickening of the stratum corneum, which is broader than thick (cf. Figs. 2.3 and 7.1). From a clinical point of view, it is characterized by circumscribed or diffuse lesions, very adherent and hard on palpation. The feeling on palpation is very peculiar because

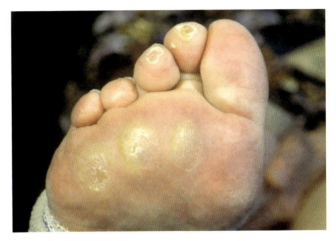

Fig. 7.1 Keratosis. Callosity. Keratosis corresponds to a thickening of the stratum corneum, which is more horizontally spread (superficially) than vertically raised (in height). In contrast, a cutaneous horn (cf. Fig. 7.2) is a keratosis that is more elevated than superficially spread. Keratosis and cutaneous horn are rough and adherent lesions, not easily dislodged and causing bleeding upon removal, as opposed to scales and crusts. In callosities, there is thickening of the stratum corneum producing a thickening, roughness, and yellow appearance of the skin. Note that the cutaneous microrelief including epidermal ridges (dermatoglyphs) is perfectly left intact, as opposed to other keratotic lesions such as plantar warts (cf. Fig. 12.55)

keratosis confers a rigid hard effect to the skin which turns out to be inflexible under finger pressure. A feeling of roughness can also be noted on rubbing. Skin exploration using the curette confirms this feeling of hardness; it is almost impossible to remove any scales.

A *cutaneous horn* is a thicker keratosis, which is more elevated than broad (Fig. 7.2).

A millimeter-wide, punctuate keratosis, covering and infiltrating the hair follicles, is called a horny plug (Fig. 7.3).

Finally, certain lesions known as porokeratoses are well demarcated and lined by a fine, keratotic collarette, which is very typical, elevated, and adherent (Fig. 7.4).

D. Lipsker, *Clinical Examination and Differential Diagnosis of Skin Lesions*, DOI 10.1007/978-2-8178-0411-8_7, © Springer-Verlag France 2013

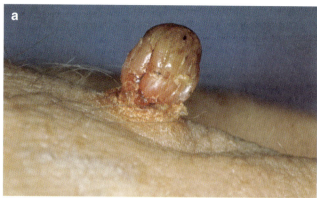

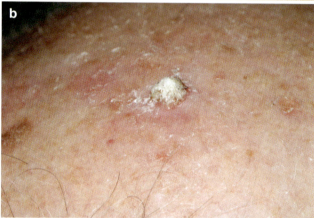

Fig. 7.2 Cutaneous horn. Warts. Actinic keratosis. (**a**) Exophytic lesion of the stratum corneum (pointing outwards) corresponding to a wart. (**b**) The horn is located on a red lesion, barely elevated and identified on its borders. The lesion is an actinic keratosis, which is a very superficial squamous cell carcinoma (cf. Chap. 13). Also note the skin of the scalp. It is red and brown and covered with numerous actinic keratoses, which illustrate the concept of field cancerization

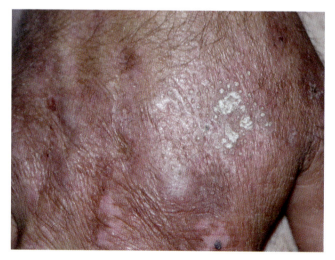

Fig. 7.3 Follicular horny plugs. Chronic lupus erythematosus. Note the follicular distribution of keratotic papules on a leukodermic plaque with erythematous borders. These horny plugs are very adherent. They are typical of chronic lupus erythematosus but may be seen in other disorders such as seborrheic keratoses or superficial pemphigus

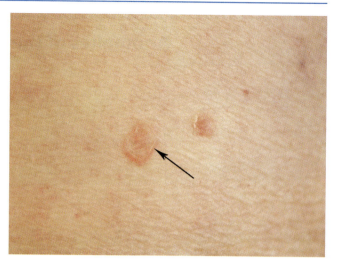

Fig. 7.4 Keratotic collarette (*arrow*). Porokeratosis. This lesion is lined with a very adherent and fine keratotic collarette, which can be felt on palpation

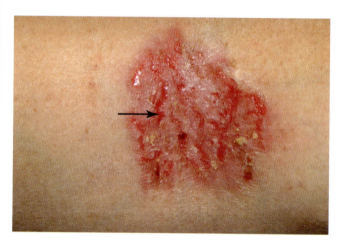

Fig. 7.5 Linear erosions on an erythematous background (*arrow*). Hailey-Hailey disease. Also note some yellow crusts, since these lesions are often (secondarily) infected. This type of linear erosion, located in a fold, is typical of Hailey-Hailey disease, which is an autosomal dominant disorder related to a defect of intercellular adhesion between epidermal keratinocytes

7.3   Skin Surface Is Absent

In this case, the skin becomes humid, oozing, serohemorrhagic, or fibrinous. These lesions are separated according to their depth. An *erosion* is a loss of the superficial part of the skin or epidermis, and it heals without leaving a scar (cf. Figs. 5.8 and 7.5). It is a humid and weeping lesion, secondarily covered by a crust and set on a bed of numerous red spots (0.1–0.2 mm) which correspond to the dermal papillae.

Excoriation is sometimes used to describe erosion occurring after a trauma, usually scratching (cf. Fig. 4.16).

A *fissure* is a fine, linear, and superficial loss of substance, without erosion of the dermis (Fig. 7.6).

An *ulceration* is a deeper loss of cutaneous substance, affecting the epidermis and the dermis and leaving a scar

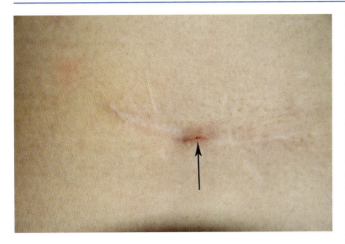

Fig. 7.6 Intracicatricial fissure (*arrow*). Fine and elongated loss of substance (<1 mm)

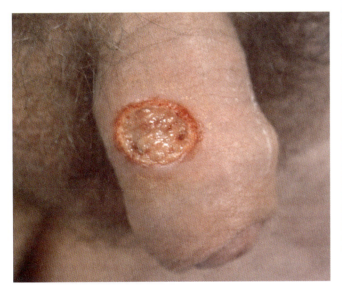

Fig. 7.7 Ulceration. Syphilitic chancre. Ulceration is a loss of cutaneous substance located deep enough to affect the epidermis and the dermis, which leaves a scar upon healing. Ulceration may be covered with a fibrinous coating, a serohemorrhagic crust (ulcerations may bleed) or a black plaque (necrosis). In this patient, there is an acute loss of substance on the penis. Note the well-defined, round borders and the fibrinous background of this ulceration. Syphilis is a classic cause of genital ulceration. These lesions are highly contagious and require that gloves be worn during examination. Palpation allows observing their induration

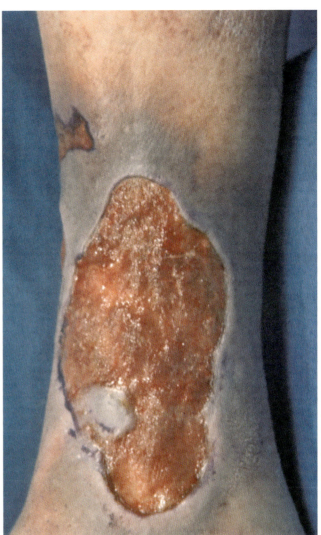

Fig. 7.8 Ulceration. Venous ulcer. An ulcer is a chronic loss of substance, without tendency to spontaneous healing and having evolved for more than a month, as in this example. Also note the brown pigmentation of the skin, a typical sign of stasis dermatitis of venous insufficiency (sometimes referred to as "dermite ocre" or ochre dermatitis)

upon healing (cf. Figs. 2.5 and 7.7). Dermal papillae are no more visible and the ulceration can be covered with a fibrinous coating, a serohemorrhagic crust (bleeding ulceration), or a black plaque (necrosis). Ulceration is described as granulating when it is covered with bright red, prominent, and much vascularized areas.

An *ulcer* is a chronic loss of substance without tendency to spontaneous healing and having evolved for more than a month (Fig. 7.8). Ulcerations occurring on pressure points produce pressure ulcers or bedsores (or decubitus ulcers).

7.4 Skin Surface Is Broken/Interrupted

Skin surface is broken by a generally round and small orifice, while the epidermis remains normally present. The *comedo* (Fig. 7.9), for example, is a millimeter-wide orifice corresponding to a visible interruption of the skin surface produced by a normal but dilated hair follicle, filled with keratin.

A *sinus tract* or a *fistula* (Fig. 7.10) is connected to the skin via an opening or cutaneous orifice of variable depth which may exude fluid.

A *rhagade* is a fine depression of less than 1 mm, without loss of substance. It can be superficial or deep and occurs on inflammatory or keratotic skin (Fig. 7.11). It is usually located in periorificial areas (labial commissures), folds, and soles.

Comedos, sinus tracts, and fistulas are nosological and not semiological terms; there is no standard semiological term to describe the gap in the skin surface.

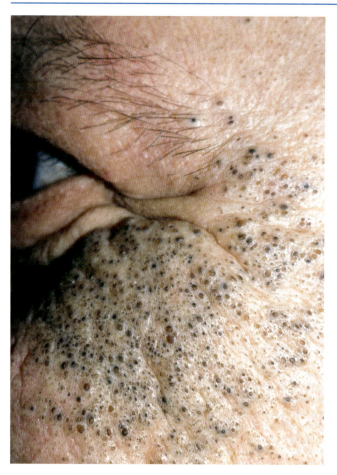

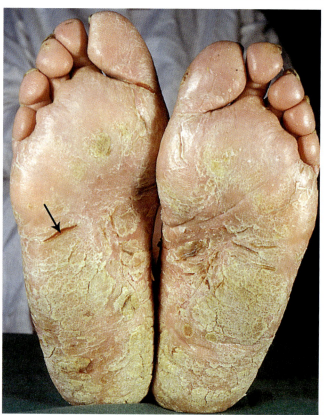

Fig. 7.11 Rhagade. Psoriasis. Linear fissures (*arrow*) seem to be breaking the stratum corneum, which is thick and yellow in this patient

Fig. 7.9 Millimeter-wide gap in the skin surface, filled with a "black spot." Comedo. Favre-Racouchot disease. It is an alteration of the skin surface, which is broken by an orifice. However, the orifice is covered by the epidermis, unlike in erosion or ulceration. Comedos are characteristic of acne; however, they may be the expression of other diseases (cf. Chap. 1, page 5), as in this example of Favre-Racouchot disease, which is a particular form of skin aging induced by sun exposure and tobacco smoking

7.5   Skin Surface Is Covered

Skin surface is covered mainly by scales and crusts.

Scales are lamellae of stratum corneum cells located at the surface of the skin (cf. Fig. 2.7). They are slightly adherent and easily removed. They are immediately visible or become apparent upon rubbing with a blunt curette. Scales can also be revealed by rubbing the skin with a black cloth. One can typically distinguish:

- Scales similar to those observed in scarlet fever (scarlatiniform) (Fig. 7.12): large shedding flaps of scales which reflect a sudden, intense, and transient production of stratum corneum. This is typical of scarlatina (scarlet fever), Kawasaki syndrome, toxic shock syndrome, recurring scarlatiniform scaled erythema Féréol-Besnier, certain drug eruptions, and final stages of several exanthemas.
- Scales forming a collarette (Fig. 7.13): thin scales, which are adherent in the periphery but not in the center and cover an inflammatory lesion (e.g., Gibert's pityriasis rosea). A collarette can also be observed in glucagonoma syndrome (necrolytic migratory erythema), superficial pemphigus syndrome, Sneddon-Wilkinson disease, candidiasis, impetigo, and syphilis.

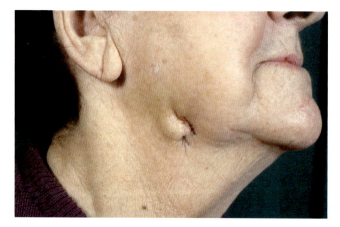

Fig. 7.10 Dental fistula. A fistula is an orifice which is connected to the skin and usually exudes fluid. This example shows a dental fistula; the collection from a dental root infection produced the nodule which is located above the orifice of the fistula

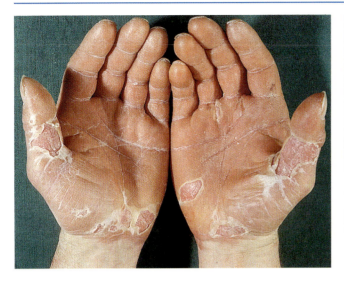

Fig. 7.12 Shedding of large scales. Scarlatiniform scaled erythema Féréol-Besnier. Very peculiar type of flaking in large shreds of skin, measuring up to several centimeters. Usually the underlying skin is then diffusely red. This type of scaling is characteristic of diseases resulting from an immune activation by a superantigen such as scarlatina, staphylococcal toxic shock syndrome, or Kawasaki disease. It appears after the acute phase of the disease and allows the retrospective diagnosis

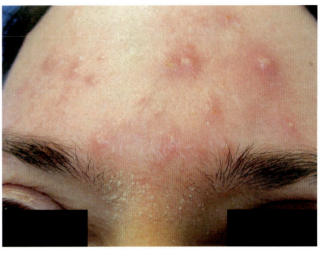

Fig. 7.14 Pityriasiform scales. Mixed facial dermatitis. Small, white, slightly adherent scales in the glabellar area. This type of scaling may occur in the course of most inflammatory dermatitis. Also note the papulopustules on the forehead. Mixed facial dermatitis combines the elements of two common types of dermatitis: usually rosacea and seborrheic dermatitis (cf. Chap. 12)

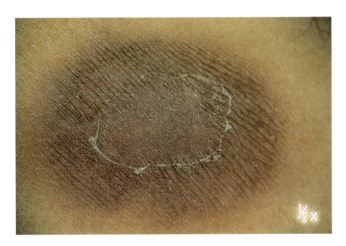

Fig. 7.13 Collarette-like scaling. This type of scaling is easily identified since scales are round and adherent in the center but not on the fringes

- Pityriasiform scales (Fig. 7.14): thin small scales, slightly adherent, of a whitish color and floury texture. They are typical of pityriasis capitis (dandruff) but can be seen in most erythematosquamous dermatoses.
- Ichthyosiform scaling (Fig. 7.14): large polygonal scales resembling fish scale. The scaly components usually break off from very dry skin, while they can sometimes be very adherent (Fig. 7.15b).
- Psoriasiform scales (Fig. 7.16): white, shiny, lamellar, silver, large, and numerous. They are typical of psoriasis and reflect parakeratosis from a histological point of view.

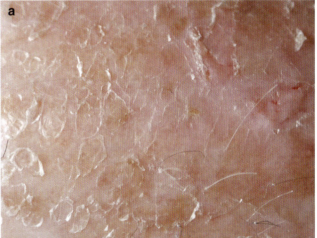

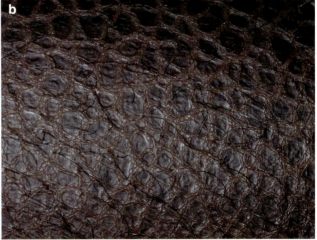

Fig. 7.15 Polygonal scales (keratosis). Ichthyosis (**a**, **b**). This appearance is sometimes described as "crocodile skin". It is characteristic of ichthyoses. Scales can be quite adherent

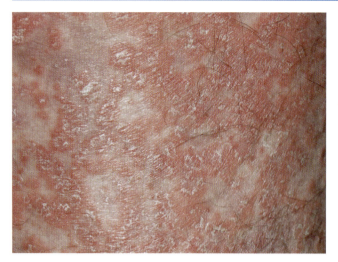

Fig. 7.16 Psoriasiform scales. Psoriasis. These scales are white, lamellar, and numerous. Rubbing with a curette causes homogeneous whitening

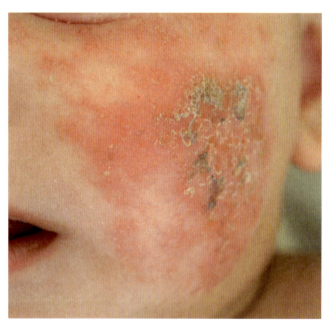

Fig. 7.17 Honey-colored crusts. Impetiginized atopic dermatitis. A crust is a concretion (i.e., solidification) of biological fluid (lymph, serosity, pus, blood) at the surface of the skin. Note the honey-yellow color of the crust, characteristic of impetigo. Erythema of the convex part of the cheek is characteristic of atopic dermatitis in infants

A *crust* is the superficial drying of exudate, secretion, necrosis, or cutaneous hemorrhage (cf. Figs. 2.8, 5.15, and 7.17). It gives a feeling of roughness on palpation. It adheres

to the lesions it covers but, unlike keratoses, it can always be removed with a curette. A crust should always be removed in order to observe the lesion beneath (ulceration, tumor, etc.).

7.6 Skin Surface Is Raised by Fluid

This applies to vesicles, bullae, or pustules, which are covered in Chap. 5. These lesions are recalled here for teaching purposes only. Indeed they are listed among alterations of the skin surface due to their physiopathological consequences (hydroelectrolytic loss, cutaneous gap).

7.7 Skin Surface Is Insensitive to All Modes

The skin is cold and becomes successively pale, blue, and black, and a groove is secondarily formed between damaged and healthy tissues. This is necrosis (cf. Figs. 2.10 and 7.18). Necrosis reflects a cutaneous infarct resulting from vascular obstruction. Gangrene and necrosis indicate a nonviable portion of cutaneous tissue which tends to be eliminated.

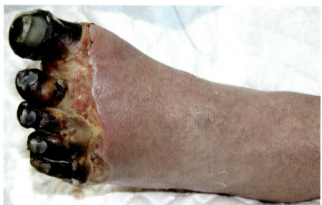

Fig. 7.18 Necrosis: black, insensitive, and cold skin. Frostbite. At the back of the necrosis, there is a fibrinous ulceration separated from healthy skin by a groove, which is always produced secondarily between viable and necrotic parts

7.8 Clinicopathological Correlations: Mechanisms

The clinicopathological correlation is usually obvious in these lesions. The precise physical examination immediately gives information about microscopic alterations, since they affect the epidermis and are directly visible. The precise description of the alterations of the lesion's surface allows predicting part of the underlying histological modifications. These alterations reflect the processes taking place in the epidermis and the superficial layer of the stratum corneum. A normal cutaneous surface confirms the absence of epidermal lesions (other than anomalies of pigmentation), indicating that the pathological process is taking place in the dermis and/or the hypodermis. When a biopsy is needed to determine the cause of an ulceration, it must be done on the border of the lesion since microscopic analysis of the loss of substance is not significant.

The main alterations of the skin surface are scaling, crusting, keratosis, erosion, ulceration, and necrosis. An alteration of the skin surface may be the only lesion present in a patient. However, it may often occur over a preexisting lesion which may or may not still be present.

The association of elementary lesions produces an actual lesional syndrome. Alterations of the skin surface allow a better description of these complex lesions, and their identification allows pathogenic and diagnostic interpretations.

The identification of primary lesions requires careful inspection and palpation. Simple techniques can be used to refine diagnosis and provide additional information.

8.1 Diascopy

This technique is performed by compressing a lesion with a transparent object (made of glass or plastic), thus "emptying" the dermal vessels (i.e., when pressure is applied, blood is forced out of the superficial blood vessels). Hence, erythemas caused by a vasoactive mediator are blanched since they are exclusively due to vasodilation, whereas redness related to purpura persists (purpura being an extravasation of red blood cells related to cutaneous hemorrhage) (cf. Fig. 4.8). This technique also enables to see the actual color of certain highly vascularized lesions, which is often obscured by the bright red color of hemoglobin (e.g., Spitz nevus usually appears red and its actual brown color is only revealed by diascopy, Fig. 8.1). Diascopy of certain lesions sometimes reveals their yellow-brown color; these lesions are known as lupoid (e.g., lupus vulgaris, sarcoidosis, Fig. 8.2).

8.2 Wood's Light Examination

This examination is done in the dark, under ultraviolet light (λ = 400 nm). Epidermal skin pigmentation is exacerbated, thus increasing the contrast between normal skin and depigmented areas (e.g., vitiligo, chemical leukoderma, piebaldism). This technique can also be used for the rapid detection of urine porphyrins which take on a pink color under Wood's light, following acidification. Finally, several infectious dermatoses are revealed by their characteristic fluorescence under Wood's light: coral

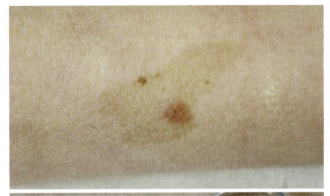
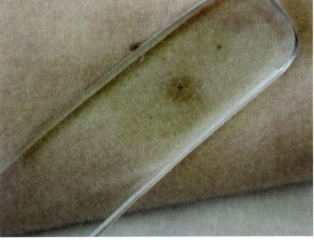

Fig. 8.1 Diascopy. Spitz Nevus. There is a red papule on a café au lait patch. The *brown color* of the papule appears only on diascopy. Multiple eruptive Spitz nevi can sometimes be found on café au lait patches

red fluorescence in erythrasma, green fluorescence in dermatophytoses caused by *Microsporum* as well as in favus, and green-yellow fluorescence in *Pseudomonas* infections. When suspecting scabies, furrows can be researched under Wood's light, after application of tetracycline or fluorescein.

D. Lipsker, *Clinical Examination and Differential Diagnosis of Skin Lesions*,
DOI 10.1007/978-2-8178-0411-8_8, © Springer-Verlag France 2013

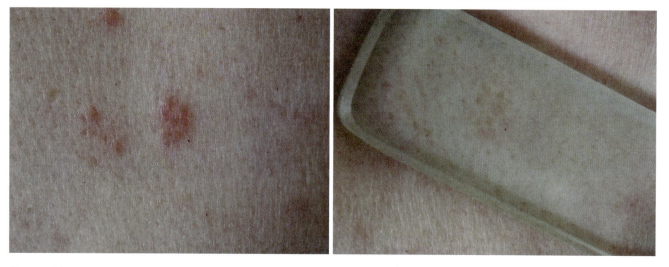

Fig. 8.2 Diascopy. Lupoid. Sarcoidosis. This erythematous papule turns out to be lupoid on diascopy, due to the fact that yellow (apple-jelly) grains present in the dermis become apparent when blood is expelled by the slide. This sign reflects a granulomatous disorder or a lymphoma

8.3   Applying Certain Substances on the Skin

Useful information can be obtained:
- Application of a drop of oil eliminates air in between scales and modifies the refractive index of keratin. This is especially useful in identifying Wickham's striae of lichen.
- Application of Indian ink, followed by rinsing, allows to identify scabies furrows without using a Wood's lamp; a felt-tip pen can also be used as the coloring agent which has penetrated the furrow persists after rinsing (cf. Fig. 12.35).

8.4   Linear Stimulation

Firm stimulation using a blunt tip enables to search for dermographism (cf. Fig. 12.20). Rubbing of certain lesions elicits an urticarial response, referred to as *Darier's sign*, which is characteristic of mastocytosis (cf. Figs. 15.69 and 15.70).

8.5   Skin Traction

Traction of normal and/or peribullous skin may cause skin detachment (Fig. 8.3): this *Nikolsky's sign* occurs in intraepidermal bullous diseases, in toxic epidermal necrolysis (Lyell's syndrome), and in certain junctional bullous diseases (such as acquired epidermolysis bullosa). A bulla which extends when vertical pressure is exerted on its top is also known to be an *Asboe-Hansen sign* and has the same significance as Nikolsky's sign.

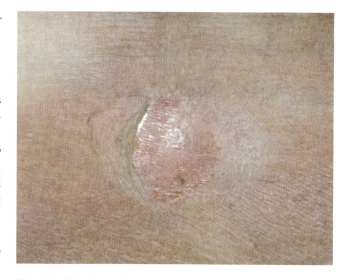

Fig. 8.3 Nikolsky's phenomenon (or sign). Stevens-Johnson syndrome. Lateral traction of the skin causes epidermal detachment. A bulla which extends when vertical pressure is exerted on its top is also known to be an Asboe-Hansen sign. It is usually an indicator of the severity of the dermatosis. Clinical examination allows to suspect the level of cleavage (intraepidermal or dermal): dry skin in case of intraepidermal detachment and moist skin in case of deeper detachment. However, this can only be ascertained by histopathological examination

8.6   Köbner and Renbök Phenomenon

The Köbner phenomenon refers to disease-specific skin lesions appearing on lines of trauma (Fig. 8.4). The Renbök phenomenon is the inverse counterpart: It refers to the case where a dermatitis does not spread on a cutaneous area already affected by another dermatitis (Fig. 8.5). The various

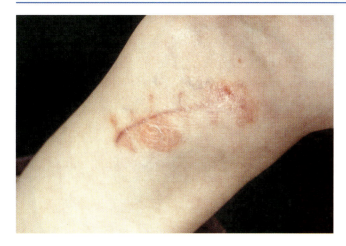

Fig. 8.4 Köbner phenomenon. Psoriasis. The disease favors traumatized cutaneous areas, as in this example, psoriasis appearing on a scar. When the disease appears on a traumatized area in a patient in whom this disorder has never been observed before, it is called a "mnémodermie de Jacquet" in the French terminology

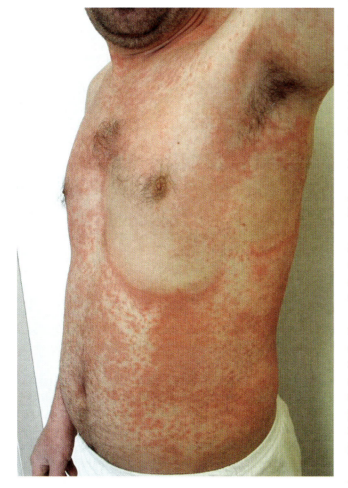

Fig. 8.5 Renbök phenomenon. Cutaneous drug reaction not spreading on areas affected by a centrifugal annular erythema. The Renbök phenomenon (reverse spelling of Köbner) is the inverse counterpart of the Köbner phenomenon. In this example, drug eruption completely avoids the areas previously affected by centrifugal annular erythema (red arciform lesions) in the area under the left breast and axilla

types of lesions that may be induced by cutaneous trauma are presented in Table 8.1.

8.7   Vertical Pressure

It enables to investigate the extent to which an edema can be depressed (pitting edema, Fig. 8.6), as well as to estimate the capillary refill time (time to recovery of normal coloration of the skin after blanching), and to investigate dermal alterations in certain raised lesions such as neurofibromas (cf. Fig. 5.8), perisudoral lipomas, piezogenic papules, or anetodermas, which are depressible. *Crepitation* can also be detected (i.e., the feeling of small air bubbles exploding under finger pressure). It reveals the presence of air in soft areas and commands an immediate etiological diagnosis in order to avoid overlooking anaerobic infections which may have dreadful prognoses.

8.8   Skin Pinching

The epidermis and dermis are movable relatively to the hypodermis. Pinching thus allows localizing hypodermal or deeper-seated lesions, over which skin folds normally. Intradermal papules such as dermatofibromas can also be localized using this technique; folding of the skin over these lesions produces dimples. Finally, pinching sometimes causes the extrusion of white, viscous material through follicular orifices (e.g., *Kreibich's sign* in follicular mucinosis, Fig. 8.7).

8.9   Scratching

Scratching of certain lesions with the nail or a blunt curette (Brocq's curette) reveals scaling, which is characteristic of psoriasis, or produces a linear purpura (e.g., amyloidosis).

Thus, in psoriasis, scratching with a Brocq's curette initially produces white-powdered scales (as when scratching a wax candle: "signe de la tache de bougie," in French terminology). Then, there is the "sign of the last removable scale," when the last suprapapillary scales are scraped off as a whole, and, finally, the Auspitz sign which consists of punctate bleeding spots as a result of removal of the epidermis and thus exposing the hypervascularized dermal papillae.

8.10   Examination with a Ten Diopter Magnifier Lens

This examination enables more precise inspection and better identification of alterations of the surface of lesions.

Table 8.1 Various types of cutaneous lesions that can be induced by a trauma

Köbner phenomenon or sign	Isomorphic response of the skin which reproduces the characteristic skin lesion of a specific disease following trauma	Examples: psoriatic plaques and papules of lichen planus reproducing exactly the traumatized area
Renbök phenomenon or sign (the inverse counterpart of the Köbner phenomenon)	Inverse isomorphic reaction: A dermatitis avoids the area already affected by another dermatitis	Example: alopecia areata avoiding a congenital nevus, a "port-wine stain" or cutaneous areas already covered by psoriasis
"Mnémodermie de Jacquet"	Köbner phenomenon appearing on a traumatized skin while patient did not yet display any sign of the disease	Example: papules of lichen planus on scratches made on the skin, prior to patient being affected by lichen
Wolf's isotopic response	Onset of a second different disease at the site of a healed disease	Example: granuloma annulare or lymphoma at the site of a zoster
Nikolsky's sign	Bullous detachment occurring on apparently normal skin when strong pressure is applied. This appears in patients affected by certain bullous disorders caused by a disruption of the inter-keratinocyte or dermo-epidermal cohesion	Examples: pemphigus, Lyell's syndrome, epidermolysis bullosa
Lichenification Accentuation of skin markings on thick and shiny skin	Caused by repeated scratching	Example: circumscribed or diffuse lichenifications

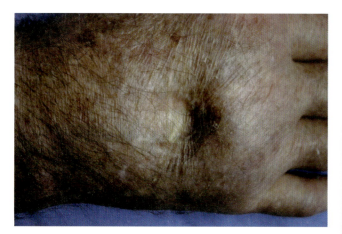

Fig. 8.6 Pitting edema (pressure with the finger induces a dimple). RS3PE (remitting seronegative symmetric synovitis with pitting edema = seronegative rheumatoid arthritis in elderly patients). This sign indicates that edema is depressible and retains the imprinted mark. This type of rheumatoid arthritis in elderly patients is usually seronegative, corticosensitive, and often reactive. It commands the investigation of cancer, blood disorders, systemic diseases, and infections

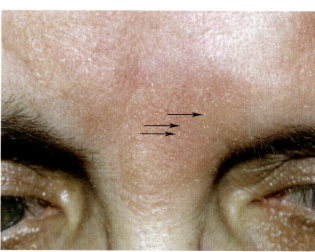

Fig. 8.7 Kreibich's sign. Follicular mucinosis. Extrusion of fine, white, mucinous material from hair follicles (*arrows*) upon pressure exerted between the thumb and index finger

8.11   Dermatoscopy

During examination of lesions by immersion or epi-illumination, application of a drop of oil or a hydroalcoholic rinsing solution allows inspection through the stratum corneum which becomes transparent. This examination is particularly interesting for pigmented lesions since it enables analysis of the epidermal pigment network.

8.12   Other Signs

Other signs, which are not explored in this book, can also be useful for diagnosis and/or understanding of pathogenesis. These are, for example:

- The flounce appearance ("signe du drapé" in French terminology): the skin of the back has large and harmonious folds (Fig. 8.8); this sign reflects cutaneous infiltration by inflammatory or tumoral cells.
- The crumbling appearance: numerous satellite lesions surrounding a larger "parent" lesion (Fig. 8.9). This is a classical sign of allergic contact dermatitis and candidiasis.
- The flowing phenomenon, where a linear erythema, potentially inducing alterations of the cutaneous surface, follows the track of an irritative or allergenic substance along the skin (Fig. 8.10).

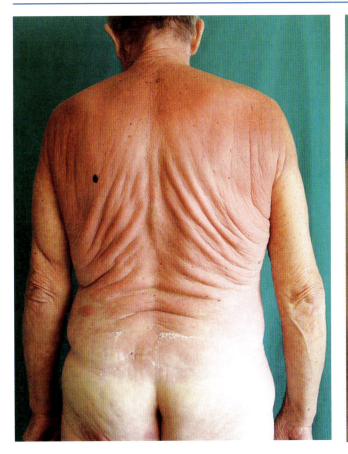

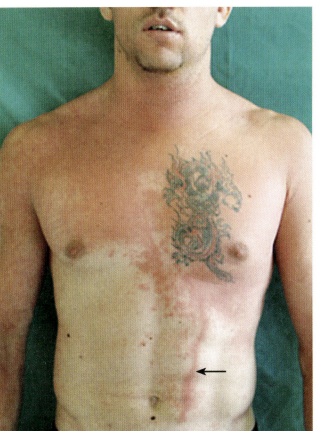

Fig. 8.8 "Flounce" appearance. Mycosis fungoides erythroderma. The skin of the back has large and harmonious folds. This sign reflects cutaneous skin infiltration by inflammatory or tumoral cells. It can be the only sign of a chronic, generalized, infiltrative dermatitis

Fig. 8.10 Flowing phenomenon (*arrow*). Contact dermatitis due to ketoprofen gel. Linear erythema, well visible under the tattoo. The dermatitis is localized on the tracks of the allergenic or irritative substance

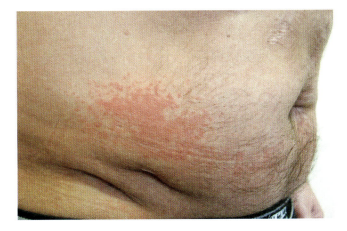

Fig. 8.9 Crumbling appearance. Allergic contact dermatitis. At the periphery of the central erythematous area, note the extension in the form of multiple, small, red lesions. This sign is highly characteristic of allergic contact dermatitis; in the case of pustular, crumbling intertrigo, candidiasis must be suspected

Configuration and Arrangement

Arrangement is the positioning of various lesions relative to each other, as opposed to configuration, which indicates the shape of an isolated primary lesion. Various types of configurations and arrangements are illustrated in Table 9.1. For example, a lesion may become annular by centrifugal extension of a single lesion (Fig. 9.1). Its configuration (shape) is then called annular. A lesion may also become annular through the confluence of different lesions which take the shape of a ring: This is called an annular arrangement (Fig. 9.2). In granuloma annulare, which is a dermatosis of unknown cause, both types of lesions described above may coexist. Linear arrangement is another type of particular

arrangement (Fig. 9.3). Its underlying mechanisms as well as certain cases of linear dermatoses are illustrated in Table 9.2.

Certain configurations have a remarkable aspect such as the target shape which has two or three concentric rings (Fig. 9.4) and immediately directs to the diagnosis of erythema multiforme. Erythema multiforme is a morphologically characteristic cutaneous reaction which can be observed in several infections and/or viral reactivations, particularly in herpes.

Table 9.1 Arrangement and configuration

Arrangement of various lesions relative to each other	Configuration (shape of an individual lesion)
Isolated	Discoid, nummular (Fig. 9.12)
Grouped	Annular (Fig. 9.1)
Clustered (cf. Fig. 2.2)	Arciform (incomplete ring) (Fig. 9.13)
Agminated (lesions that are grouped in a specific anatomical area) (Fig. 9.5)	Target-shaped (Fig. 9.4)
Corymbiform (lesions that are grouped around a central lesion)	Digitiform (finger-shaped) (Fig. 9.14)
Annular (Fig. 9.2)	Linear (Fig. 9.3)
Arciform (Fig. 9.6)	Stellar (Fig. 9.15)
Petaloid (confluence of round, full lesions, as opposed to the annular confluence of round lesions with a healing center, producing polycyclic lesions) (Fig. 9.7)	Oval
Polycyclic (Fig. 9.8)	Serpiginous (cf. Fig. 4.27)
Linear (Fig. 9.9)	Reticulated (cf. Fig. 3.10)
Serpiginous (cf. Fig. 4.25a)	Cribriform (forms a grid) (cf. Fig. 2.5)
Reticulated (forms a network) (Figs. 9.10 and 9.11)	

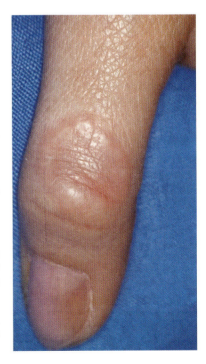

Fig. 9.1 Annular configuration. Granuloma annulare. Annular plaque on the back of the thumb, displaying a normal center and papular border, without alteration of the cutaneous surface. The cutaneous surface is unaltered, thus ruling out dermatophytosis, which is a highly prevalent annular dermatitis and usually has scaling borders (cf. Fig. 12.36). Granuloma annulare is an inflammatory skin disease of unknown cause

D. Lipsker, *Clinical Examination and Differential Diagnosis of Skin Lesions*, DOI 10.1007/978-2-8178-0411-8_9, © Springer-Verlag France 2013

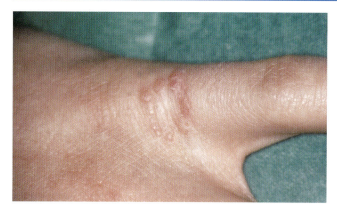

Fig. 9.2 Annular arrangement. Wart. Here, it is an annular arrangement and not a configuration. Indeed, the ring shape is produced by the confluence of several lesions. Compare with Fig. 9.1, where the lesion has an annular shape

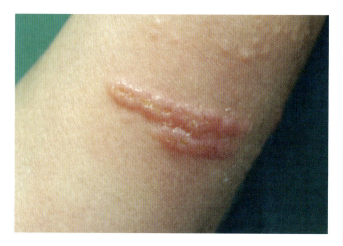

Fig. 9.3 Linearity. Chemical burn by exposure to sodium hydroxide solution. Linearity almost always reflects an exogenous cause. In this example, the linear configuration is more important diagnostically than the primary lesion, which is a partially crusting, edematous plaque

Table 9.2 Mechanisms and examples of linear dermatoses

Mechanisms	Examples/comments
Related to blood vessels or lymph vessels (Fig. 9.16)	Superficial thrombophlebitis, lymphangitis (septic, neoplastic, inflammatory, etc.), linear but broken dissemination along a lymphatic vessel (sporotrichoid), etc.
Along the course of a nerve segment (resembles a distribution) (Fig. 9.17)	Zoster, post-zoster eruption (Wolf's isotopic response): pseudolymphoma, lymphoma, granuloma annulare, lichen, eruptive epidermoid cysts, granulomatous folliculitis, etc.
Along Blaschko lines (Figs. 9.18 and 9.19)	These lines trace the migration of cutaneous stem cells during embryogenesis
Along skin lines (Figs. 9.20 and 9.21)	*Sherrington's lines:* These lines separate cutaneous areas corresponding to different medullar segments. Certain pigmentary demarcation lines (type A) could be an example. *Voigt's lines:* These lines stand in between cutaneous fields of peripheral nerves
	Segmental neurofibromatosis is an example

Table 9.2 (continued)

Mechanisms	Examples/comments
	Langer's lines (cleavage lines): These lines are caused by mechanical traction. They indicate the direction for cutaneous incision
	Wallace's lines: These lines are virtual demarcations between the palm and the back of the hand and between the sole and the back of the foot. They explain the sharp demarcation of several inflammatory dermatoses at extremities
Caused by an external factor (mechanical, chemical, thermal, infectious [sting, bite, etc.], etc.) (Figs. 9.3, 9.21, and 9.22)	Numerous
	When observing linearity and, generally speaking, any geometrical or unusual eruption, an external and/or mechanical cause must be suspected first and foremost, irrespective of the nature of the clinical and histopathological lesions
Others: unknown mechanism (Figs. 9.23 and 9.24).	Linear cord in interstitial granulomatous dermatitis
	Zebra-like stripes in dermatomyositis
	Flagellated pigmentation caused by bleomycin, following consumption of shiitake mushroom, etc.

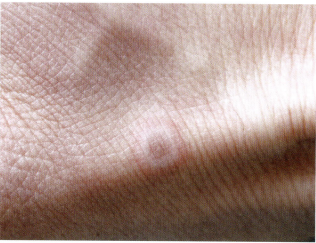

Fig. 9.4 Target-shaped. Erythema multiforme. Typical target-shaped lesions are determined by two criteria: the lesion is palpable and there are at least two concentric rings. This type of lesion highly suggests erythema multiforme, although it is not specific to the disease

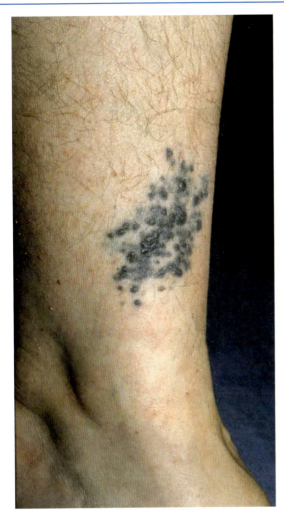

Fig. 9.5 Agminated. Blue nevus. The term "agminated" indicates grouped lesions, located close to each other

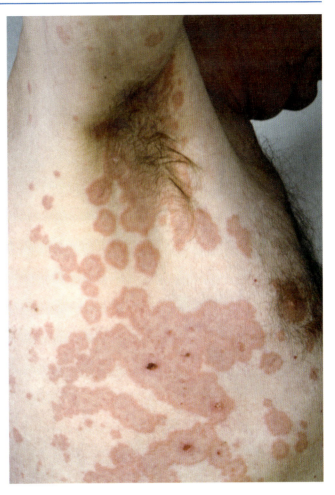

Fig. 9.7 Petaloid. Linear IgA dermatosis. The confluence of nummular lesions (full, round lesions, without central clearing) produces a petaloid appearance, as opposed to the confluence of annular lesions with central clearing, which produce a polycyclic appearance (cf. Fig. 9.8)

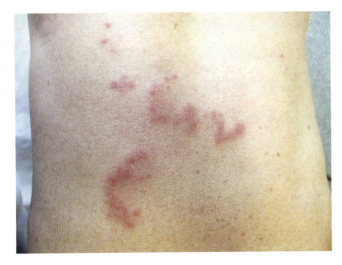

Fig. 9.6 Arciform erythematous plaques. Cutaneous lupus erythematosus (Jessner's benign lymphocytic infiltration of the skin). These lesions form incomplete rings

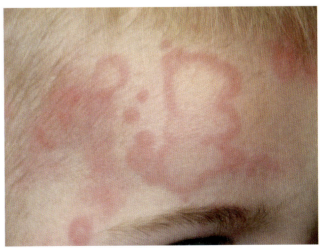

Fig. 9.8 Polycyclic. Urticaria. Confluence of annular lesions

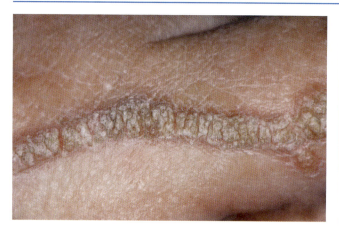

Fig. 9.9 Linearity. Wart. Köbner phenomenon. This example shows a linear warty lesion resulting from the confluence of warts. This has been induced by scratching (Köbner phenomenon, cf. Chap. 8), which explains the linearity

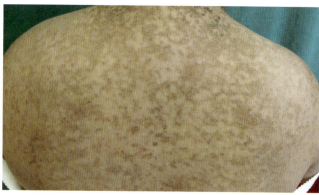

Fig. 9.11 Reticulated. Gougerot-Carteaud syndrome. In this dermatosis, the primary lesion is a keratotic brown papule which confluates over the trunk and forms a network, hence its other denomination: confluent and reticulate papillomatosis

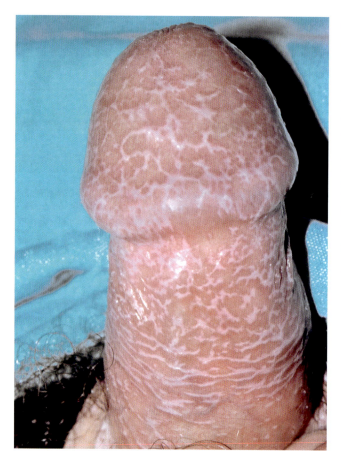

Fig. 9.10 Reticulated. Lichen. Note the leukokeratotic white lines forming a grid (network) on the glans and shaft. This example shows Wickham's striae, pathognomonic of lichen

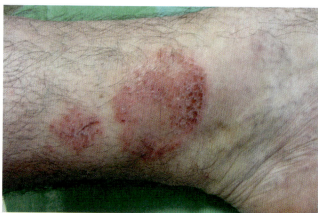

Fig. 9.12 Nummular. Stasis dermatitis. The term nummular indicates coin-shaped lesions. This example shows nummular plaques in the perimalleolar area of complex pathogenesis in the context of stasis dermatitis of venous insufficiency

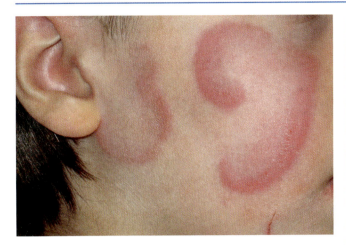

Fig. 9.13 Arciform configuration. Annular erythema in Sjögren syndrome (a dermal variant of lupus erythematosus). These lesions result from progressive centrifugal extension

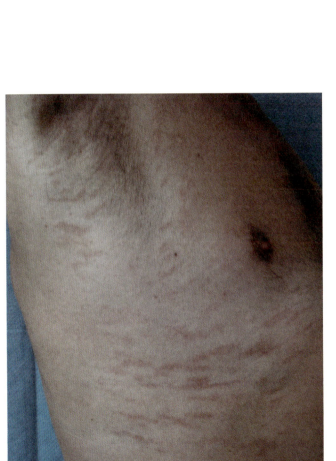

Fig. 9.14 Digitate (finger-shaped) configuration. Small plaque parapsoriasis (mycosis fungoides). Digitate means that the lesion has the shape of a finger

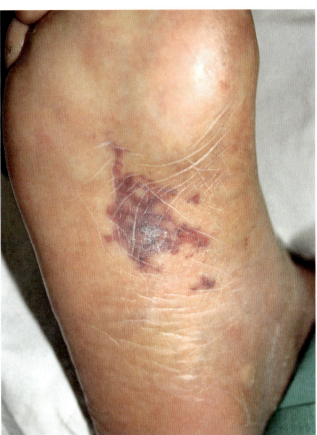

Fig. 9.15 Reticulated and stellar purpura. A reticulated and stellar (in the shape of a star) purpura always reflects a thrombosing vasculopathy and must be considered as a medical emergency

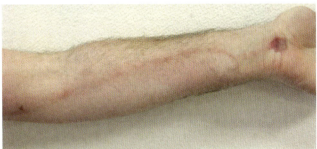

Fig. 9.16 Linearity. Lymphangitis following insect bite. This is a linear, more or less curvy erythema, which follows the course of a lymphatic vessel. It corresponds to a linearity which is anatomically determined

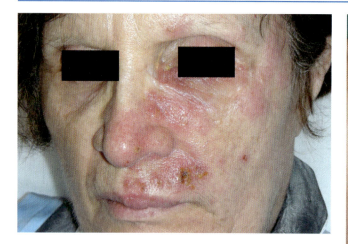

Fig. 9.17 Metameric distribution. V2 Zoster. This distribution is anatomically determined along a metamere

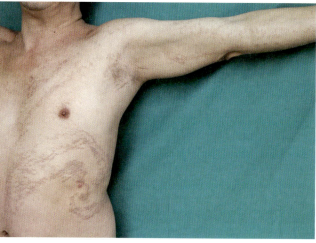

Fig. 9.19 Blaschko lines (thin). Adult Blaschko dermatitis. Blaschko dermatitis is of unknown cause and may be triggered by one or more viral infections or reactivations, i.e., a paraviral disease. Genetic mosaïcism probably contributes to the pathogenesis of inflammatory polygenic diseases distributed along these lines

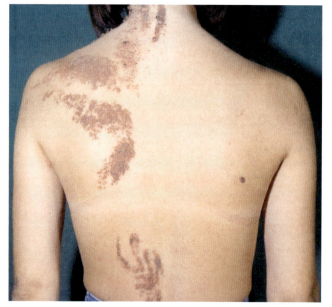

Fig. 9.18 Blaschko lines (thick). Verrucous nevus. Very unusual linear and curvy arrangement of the embryonic migration lines of cutaneous stem cells. Most monogenic and some polygenic diseases can be located along these lines known as Blaschko lines in honor of the Berliner dermatologist who first described them

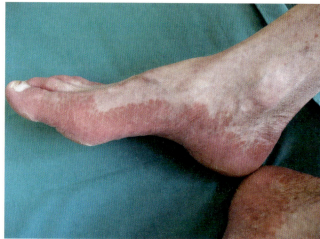

Fig. 9.20 Wallace's line. This line is a virtual demarcation between the palm and the back of the hand and between the sole and the back of the foot. These lines explain the sharp demarcation of dermatoses at extremities, as in this example of Sézary's syndrome

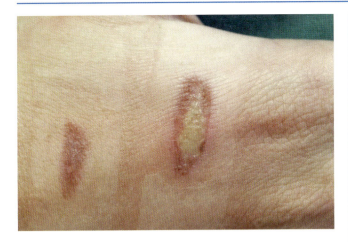

Fig. 9.21 Linearity. External cause. Erosive and ulcerated erythema, which has become fibrinous following thermal injury

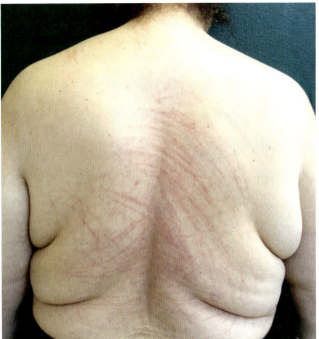

Fig. 9.23 Zebra-like or flagellated erythema. Dermatomyositis. Very unusual and rare endogenous linearity found in dermatomyositis (completely unknown mechanism) and in some intoxications (shiitake mushrooms, drugs). Depending on the context, this appearance is almost pathognomonic

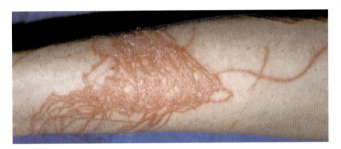

Fig. 9.22 Linearity with the configuration of a "ball of yarn." Jellyfish burn. Linearity must always suggest an external cause, as in this example of jellyfish burn

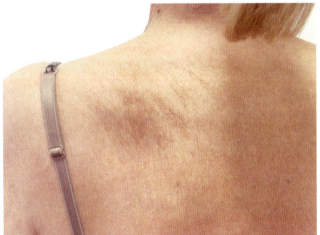

Fig. 9.24 Linear and flagellated pigmentation. Cutaneous drug reaction to bleomycin

The distribution or extension of a dermatosis must always be emphasized. The disease may be localized (single, isolated lesion) (Fig. 10.1), segmental or regional (Fig. 10.2), diffused or generalized (Fig. 10.3), or universal (Fig. 10.4).

Certain distributions have a remarkable aspect and their identification requires experience. A particular distribution may reflect the exposure of uncovered skin to a pathogen present in the environment, or to the sun. Therefore, these dermatoses will be located mainly on exposed areas: face, neck, neckline, and back of the hands and/or forearms (Figs. 10.5, 10.6, and 10.7). It may be difficult to distinguish a dermatitis caused by an airborne agent from a photoinduced dermatitis. Certain signs may be of help: the airborne agent will tend to accumulate in the exposed cutaneous folds such as the palpebral or retroauricular folds which are naturally photo protected. The airborne dermatitis will thus affect these areas which are not involved in photoinduced dermatitis. Likewise, the anterior cervical area located below the chin is naturally protected from sun exposure, i.e., the submental triangle, which will remain clear in photosensitive

dermatitis (Fig. 10.8). Distribution also gives an indication about the underlying mechanism of a lesion: a very sharp demarcation, as if traced using a ruler, is typically found in phototoxic dermatitis (Fig. 10.9), while imprecise demarcation is characteristic of photoallergic dermatitis and photoaggravated disorders (Figs. 10.5 and 10.8).

A particular distribution may also result from anatomical characteristics of the skin. For example, certain disorders

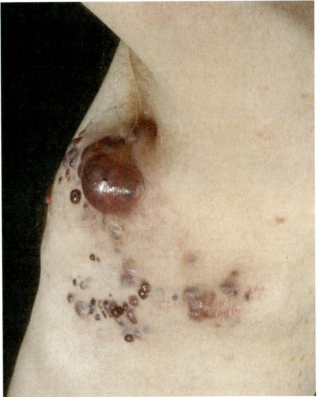

Fig. 10.2 Regional distribution. Regional cutaneous metastases in a patient with melanoma. The regional distribution may be due to several mechanisms such as the exposure of a limited cutaneous area to a pathogen, or the correspondence to an area of lymphatic drainage (as in this example), or to a metamere

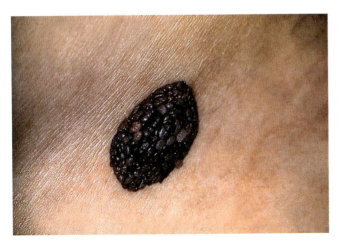

Fig. 10.1 Localized distribution. Tuberous nevus. Single lesion occurring on a very localized anatomical area. It is the case in all tumoral lesions but also in several infectious diseases. Inflammatory dermatoses such as psoriasis may be localized, segmental, diffused, or generalized

D. Lipsker, *Clinical Examination and Differential Diagnosis of Skin Lesions,*
DOI 10.1007/978-2-8178-0411-8_10, © Springer-Verlag France 2013

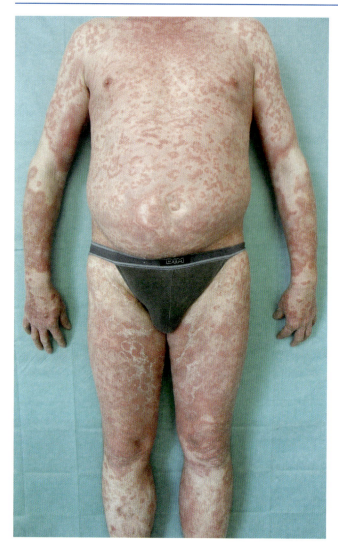

Fig. 10.3 Generalized distribution. Psoriasis. In this example, every segment of the body was affected by psoriasis. However, lesions are not confluent and the distribution is not universal, as could be the case in psoriatic erythroderma

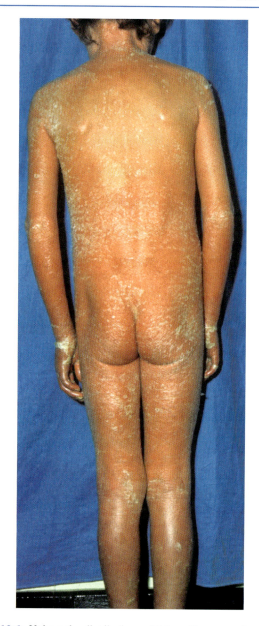

Fig. 10.4 Universal distribution. Ichthyosiform erythroderma. The entire skin is affected, including the palms and soles

are located in areas of the skin containing sebaceous glands, such as the scalp, the eyebrow area, the glabella, the nasolabial folds, and the presternal area (Fig. 10.10, and cf. Chap. 12, Seborrheic dermatitis). Other disorders affect the apocrine sweat glands which are present only in axilla, areola, and perineum. Some dermatoses are located electively on pilosebaceous follicles (Fig. 10.11).

Certain distributions indicate the presence of underlying anatomical structures, such as dermatoses occurring along the course of peripheral nerves, nerve segments, veins, or lymph vessels (cf. Table 9.2). In case of any localized inflammatory dermatosis, the underlying anatomical structures must be taken into account in order not to overlook a possible and potentially serious cutaneous inflammation, contiguous to one of these structures (bone, joint, sinus, etc.)

(cf. Inflammation by contiguity or contiguous inflammation of the skin, Chap. 15).

Certain distributions are noticeable but do not correspond to any anatomical structure that can be individualized. These dermatoses occur along Blaschko lines (cf. Table 9.2). They are generally invisible and only become apparent in certain diseases which electively occur on these specific locations. These lines reflect migration of skin cells during embryonic development. The topography of these lines is illustrated in Fig. 10.12. The identification of these noteworthy distributions often helps greatly in differential diagnosis.

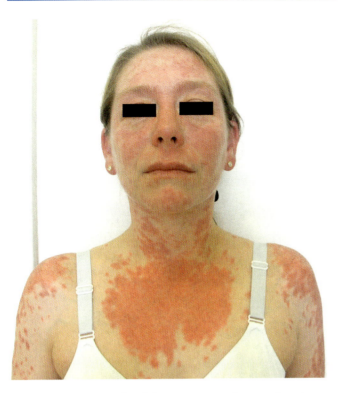

Fig. 10.5 Photodistribution. Subacute cutaneous lupus erythematosus. Lesions are predominantly located on areas exposed to ultraviolet radiation: face and neckline. Lupus erythematosus belongs to the group of photo-triggered and/or photoaggravated diseases

Finally, some dermatoses have a very characteristic distribution as, for example, the involvement of elbows and knees in psoriasis, but this is outside the scope of this book.

Table 10.1 presents a synthesis of the extensions and characteristics of dermatoses.

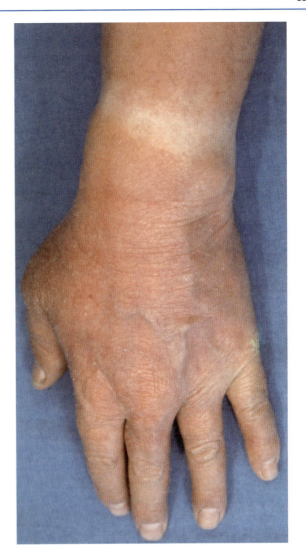

Fig. 10.6 Photodistribution. Polymorphous light eruption. Note the avoidance of the skin area protected by the watch

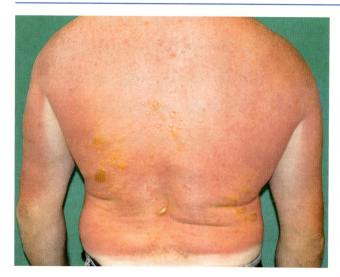

Fig. 10.7 Photodistribution. Actinic erythema (sunburn). This patient was bare chested and subjected to direct sunlight for an extended period of time; this is a severe sunburn with bullae indicating superficial second-degree burns. Note below the very sharp demarcation between the affected skin and the area protected by the pants, as well as the avoidance of naturally less exposed areas on the anteromedial part of the forearms and arms

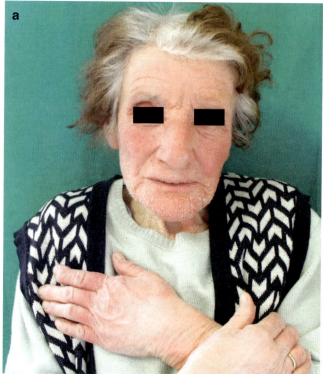

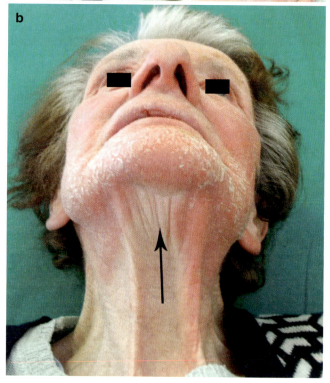

Fig. 10.8 Photodistribution (**a**, **b**). Contact dermatitis photoaggravated by topical chlorproethazine (contained in Neuriplège). Lesions are located on exposed areas of the palms and back of the hands. The avoidance of the submental triangle (**b** *Arrow*) indicates photoinduction (or aggravation). The imprecise limitation between healthy and injured skin and the extension beyond strictly photo-protected areas point to a photoallergic rather than phototoxic dermatitis

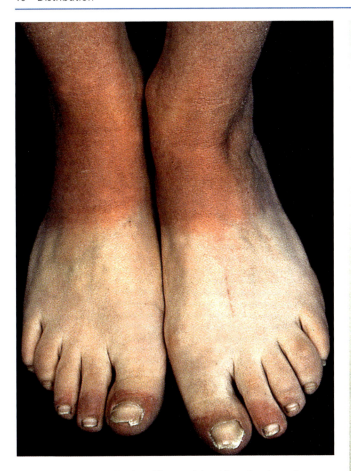

Fig. 10.9 Photodistribution. Phototoxicity. Note the sharp demarcation between affected and healthy skin, as if traced using a ruler. This type of demarcation is always an indication of the direct effect of UVs and therefore a direct phototoxic mechanism, not a photoallergic reaction

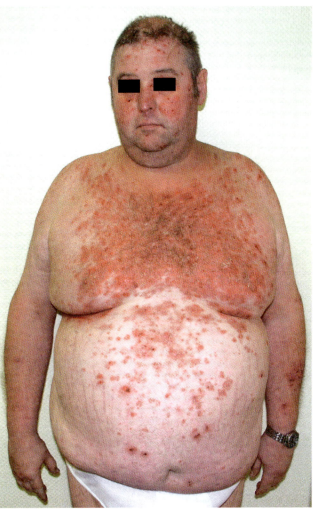

Fig. 10.10 Seborrheic distribution. Superficial pemphigus (seborrheic pemphigus). Note the particular distribution which is predominant in areas rich in sebaceous glands: face, particularly nose; scalp; torso, particularly presternal area

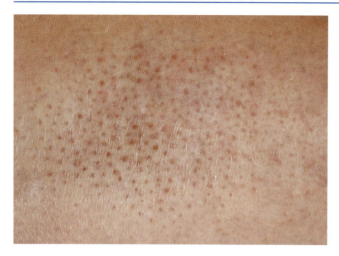

Fig. 10.11 Follicular distribution. Mycosis fungoides. Equidistant millimeter-wide papules, electively located at the emergence of pilosebaceous follicles: pilotropism. There is a pilotropic variant of this cutaneous T cell lymphoma

Table 10.1 Distribution of a dermatosis

Extension	Characteristic
Localized (folds, palms and soles, buttocks, joint surface, genital parts, characteristic, etc.) (Figs. 10.1 and 10.13)	Photodistribution (Figs. 10.5, 10.6, 10.7, 10.8, and 10.9)
Regional (Fig. 10.2)	Areas subjected to pressure points, friction, airborne substances, etc.
Generalized (Fig. 10.3)	Follicular distribution (Fig. 10.11)
Universal (Fig. 10.4)	Distribution in seborrheic areas (Fig. 10.10)
	Distribution in apocrine areas
	Anatomically determined distribution: segmental (cf. Fig. 9.17), along a blood vessel, a lymph vessel (cf. Fig. 9.16), cartilaginous areas (e.g., chondritis, Fig. 10.14), etc.
	Blaschkolinear distribution (cf. Figs. 9.18 and 9.19)
	"Endogenous" distribution (symmetrical, simultaneous affection of several folds, Fig. 10.15)
	Areas of involvement that are typical of certain dermatoses (psoriasis, lichen, scabies, secondary syphilis, atopic dermatitis, dermatitis herpetiformis, etc.)

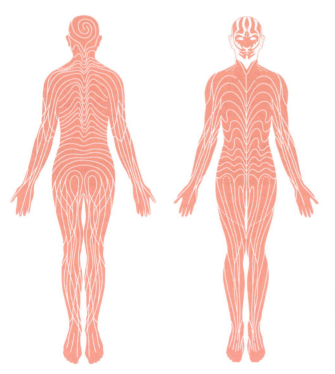

Fig. 10.12 Blaschko lines. Blaschko's original drawings complete with scalp lines according to Happle et al.

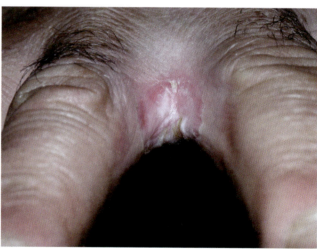

Fig. 10.13 Localized distribution occurring in a fold (interdigital). Candidiasis. Erythema occurring in a fold is also called intertrigo. Interdigital intertrigo is often caused by candidiasis

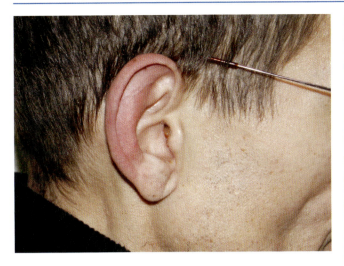

Fig. 10.14 Erythema next to the cartilaginous portion of the ear. Chondritis. Crohn's disease. Note the erythematous affection of the pinna and avoidance of the lobule, characteristic of auricular chondritis

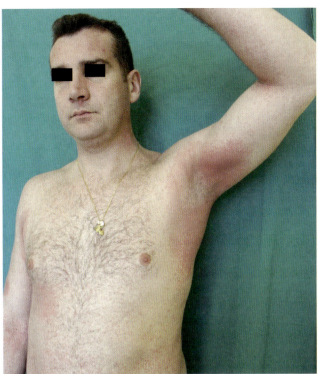

Fig. 10.15 Simultaneous affection of several folds (ptychotropism). Cutaneous drug reaction (SDRIFE: Symmetrical Drug-Related Intertriginous and Flexural Exanthema). The simultaneous affection of several folds indicates an endogenous disorder. Cutaneous drug reactions are a possible cause

Synopsis

11

Features that must be part of the description of a primary lesion are listed in Box 11.1. When a patient has several lesions, their distribution must be specified as well as a possibly notable arrangement. It is essential to identify and describe all lesions present and to record their evolution (dynamism). Thus, for example, in chickenpox, primary lesions manifest as vesicles with a cutaneomucosal distribution and no particular configuration. These lesions evolve towards umbilication and crusting, through several asynchronous flares.

Box 11.1 Descriptive Features of a Dermatological Lesion

Nature of the primary lesion

Size of the primary lesion

Disposition, configuration, and demarcations of the primary lesion

    Shape and configuration: round, oval, polygonal, target shaped, annular, linear, etc.

    Relief: flat, domed, sessile, pediculate, acuminate, umbilication, lobulated, etc.

    Demarcations: well defined, not very well defined

    Symmetry

    Regularity

Color of the lesion and effect of diascopy

Anomalies of the cutaneous surface

Consistence of the lesion

    Normal (comparable to healthy skin)

    Soft

    Firm

    Rough

    Elastic, renitent (resistant to finger pressure)

    Hard

    Depressible

    Fluctuating

Depth of the lesion

Temperature and sensitivity

D. Lipsker, *Clinical Examination and Differential Diagnosis of Skin Lesions*,
DOI 10.1007/978-2-8178-0411-8_11, © Springer-Verlag France 2013

Part II

Nosology

This section illustrates cutaneous signs of various disorders which are considered to be of significant importance.

These include signs of diseases which are potentially life threatening and whose identification entails application of a specific treatment.

These include commonly found dermatoses, encountered by every clinician, as well as cutaneous tumors. Some cutaneous tumors are very common and occur in almost every human being, while others are less frequent but are nevertheless illustrated here as they may be life threatening if not diagnosed early.

Cutaneous signs of certain general diseases are also presented in this chapter.

Common Dermatoses

12.1 Acne

Comedos, microcysts, red papules, and papulopustules (Figs. 12.1 and 12.2). Lesions are located on the face, particularly the jugal areas and the forehead, as well as the back. The comedo ("black spot" (white arrow)) and the microcyst (black arrow) are the most characteristic primary lesions of acne. The diagnosis of acne cannot be established without the presence of at least one of these two lesions, especially since papules and papulopustules are also present in rosacea, which is another prevalent facial dermatosis (cf. Figs. 12.3 and 12.4).

12.2 Rosacea

Midfacial erythema with telangiectasia, which spares the "mobile" areas of the face such as the eyelids and the circumoral area (Fig. 12.3). Papules, pustules, and papulopustules can appear on the facial erythema (Fig. 12.4). Comedos and microcysts are absent, as opposed to acne (cf. Figs. 12.1 and 12.2).

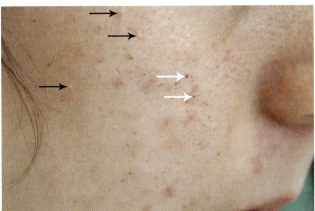

Fig. 12.1

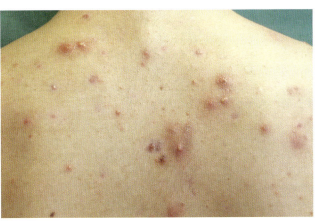

Fig. 12.2

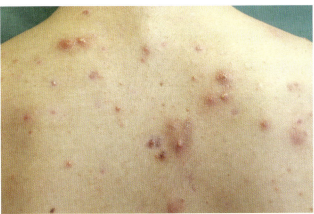

Fig. 12.3

D. Lipsker, *Clinical Examination and Differential Diagnosis of Skin Lesions*,
DOI 10.1007/978-2-8178-0411-8_12, © Springer-Verlag France 2013

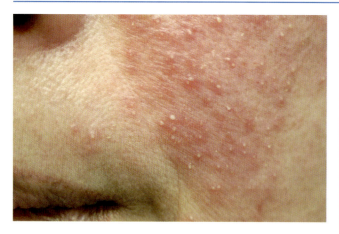

Fig. 12.4

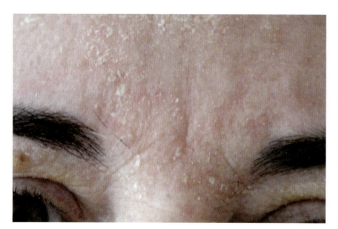

Fig. 12.5

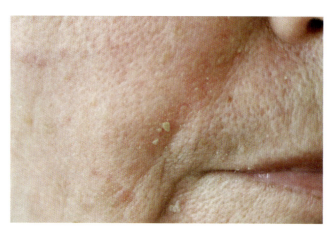

Fig. 12.6

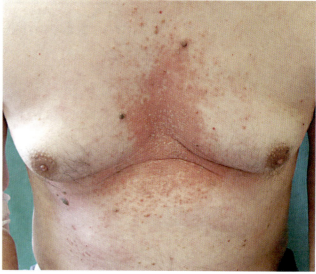

Fig. 12.7

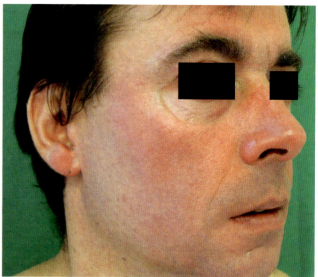

Fig. 12.8

(Fig. 12.8): This entity is known in the French nosology under the designation of mixed dermatitis of the face.

12.4 Atopic Dermatitis

Erythema of the cheeks and more generally of convex areas, in infants under 6 months (Fig. 12.9). Scaly erythema of the folds, more or less lichenified and excoriated, in adults and infants older than 6 months (Fig. 12.10). The skin is usually dry (xerosis) and the accentuation of the inferior palpebral folds is typical (Dennie-Morgan sign: double inferior palpebral fold (arrow), Fig. 12.11). Herpetic superinfection is frequent. It can be localized (Fig. 12.12; note the grouped and dried vesicles) or sometimes generalized and febrile. In

12.3 Seborrheic Dermatitis

Recurring scaly erythema, predominant in areas rich in sebum: hairline, glabella, nasolabial folds, and presternal area (Figs. 12.5–12.7).

Some patients will have lesions characteristic of both seborrheic dermatitis and rosacea at the same time

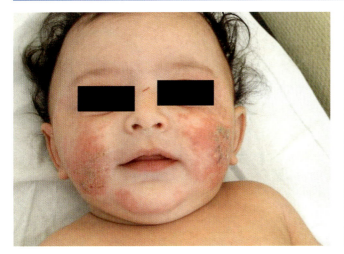

Fig. 12.9

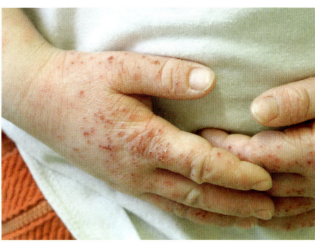

Fig. 12.12

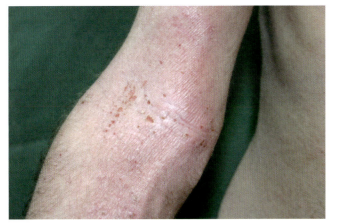

Fig. 12.10

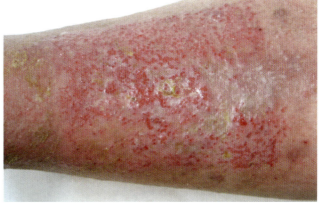

Fig. 12.13

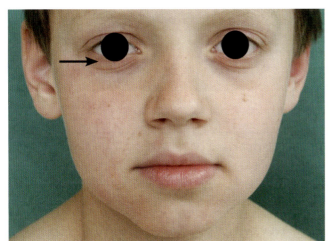

Fig. 12.11

the latter case, it is called the Kaposi-Juliusberg's syndrome, which is a life-threatening condition.

12.5 Allergic Contact Dermatitis (Eczema)

Erosive, oozing, and/or crusting erythema (Figs. 12.13, 12.14, and 12.15). Acute eczema progresses through the following stages: erythema, vesicle, oozing, and crusting. Chronic forms are erythematous, scaly, and dry (Fig. 12.16). There are several variants: bullous (Fig. 12.17), edematous, pustular (cf. Fig. 5.14), etc. Significant pruritus is present in all stages. In contact dermatitis caused by hair dye, the upper part of the face is highly edematous (Fig. 12.18) and can easily be mistaken with angioedema (urticaria of deeper skin tissues, Quincke's edema).

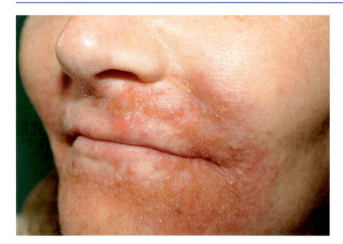

Fig. 12.14

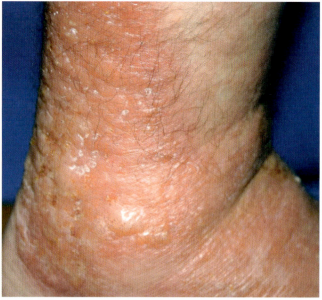

Fig. 12.17

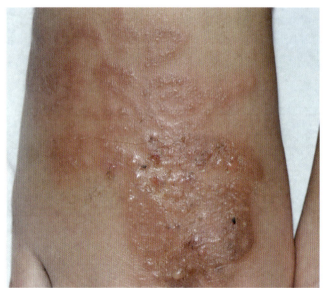

Fig. 12.15

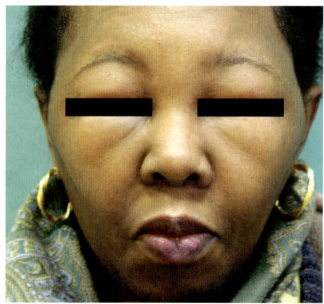

Fig. 12.18

12.6   Urticaria

Urticaria is a rash of sudden onset consisting of papules and red, edematous plaques (Fig. 12.19), mostly evanescent and pruritic. The latter semiological features are anamnestic elements and allow establishing diagnosis during history taking. In the absence of these features, it can be difficult to distinguish urticaria and maculopapular exanthema. It must be kept in mind that urticaria can be one of the manifestations of a serious anaphylactic reaction. In case of chronic urticaria, lesions can sometimes be reproduced by rubbing the skin with a blunt tip, which induces erythema + edema + pruritus. This is known as dermographism (Fig. 12.20).

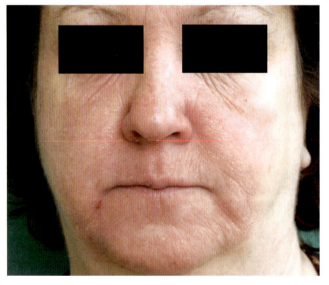

Fig. 12.16

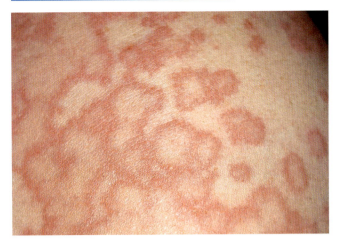

Fig. 12.19

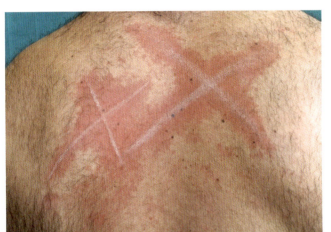

Fig. 12.20

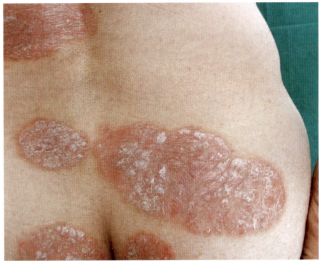

Fig. 12.21

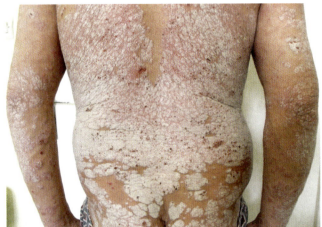

Fig. 12.22

12.7 Psoriasis

Well-defined erythematous and scaly plaques (Fig. 12.21), even when confluent (Fig. 12.22). Psoriasis is a very common dermatosis, affecting around 2 % of the population. It comprises of several clinical expressions which will not all be covered in this book. The plaque form illustrated here is the most common. The most initial lesion of common psoriasis is an erythematous macule (Fig. 12.23) which rapidly becomes scaly and infiltrated; in folds, psoriasis usually persists as an erythematous macule (intertrigo, Fig. 12.24). The sharp demarcation of the lesions is characteristic and allows diagnosis even on dark skin, where erythema is difficult to observe (Fig. 12.25).

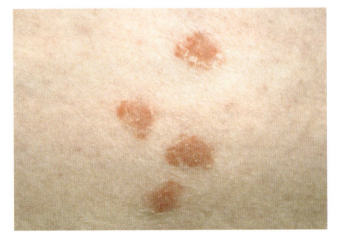

Fig. 12.23

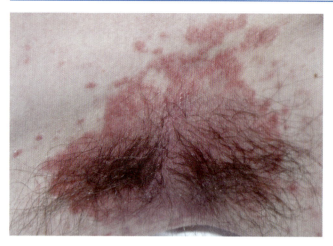

Fig. 12.24

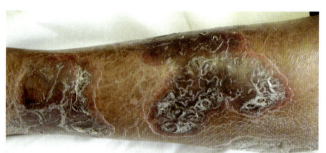

Fig. 12.25

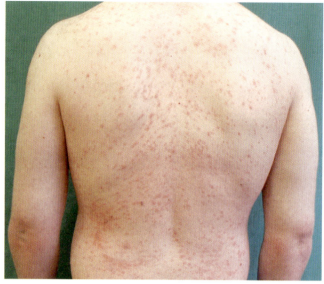

Fig. 12.26

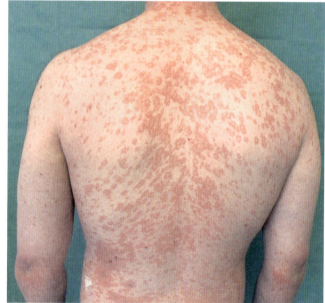

Fig. 12.27

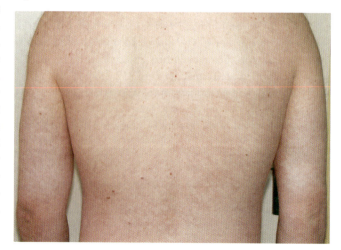

Fig. 12.28

12.8   Cutaneous Drug Reactions (CDR)

Clinical expressions of CDR are too numerous to be covered in this book. Almost all dermatoses (urticaria, pemphigoid, lichen, psoriasis, etc.) can be induced or aggravated by drugs. Clinicians should always bear this possibility in mind. Likewise, CDR has no specific morphological appearance, except for fixed drug eruption (cf. Fig. 3.9), which is quite specifically associated with exposure to certain drugs. The most serious forms of CDR are illustrated in Chap. 14. The most common dermatological expression of a cutaneous drug reaction is a maculopapular exanthema; Figs. 12.26, 12.27, and 12.28 show the progression in time of an exanthema caused by sulfamethoxazole trimethoprim (Bactrim®) (respectively days 2, 4, and 9 following the onset of the rash and the discontinuation of treatment). Initial involvement of folds is characteristic (cf. Fig. 10.15); the baboon syndrome – almost always caused by a drug – is a good example, since it shows a severe affection of the intergluteal fold and of the buttocks, which explains its denomination (Fig. 12.29).

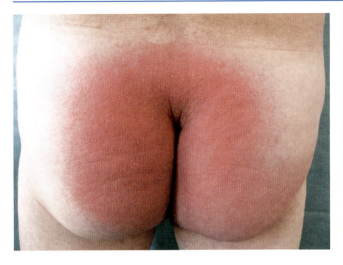

Fig. 12.29

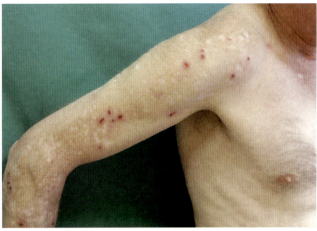

Fig. 12.31

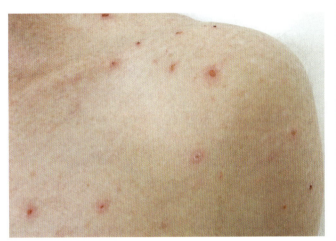

Fig. 12.30

12.9 Pruritus and Scratching

Excoriated lesions (Figs. 12.30 and 12.31). Pruritus is caused by several cutaneous and extracutaneous diseases. Schematically outlined, three situations can be identified:

- It may be a pruritic dermatosis (e.g., scabies, lichen), in which case the specific lesions enabling to identify this dermatosis must be carefully searched.
- Pruritus can also be the manifestation of a systemic disease (e.g., lymphoma, polycythemia, thyroid dysfunction, parasitosis, hypereosinophilic syndrome, renal impairment, hepatocellular insufficiency, some chronic viral infections like hepatitis C or HIV, or induced by some drugs).
- Often, no cause can be identified and pruritus is then attributed to old age (senile pruritus), to psychological factors (psychogenic pruritus), etc.

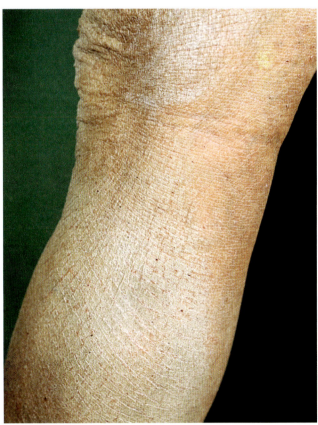

Fig. 12.32

Regardless of its cause, pruritus may lead to various cutaneous lesions as a result of the associated scratching. These lesions must be identified so as not to be given a wrong etiological significance. The lesions are excoriated papules evolving into hyper- or hypopigmented scars (Figs. 12.30 and 12.31), thickened and marked skin (lichenification, Fig. 12.32 and cf. Fig. 4.16), and sometimes firm nodules, very hard on palpation, in the context of prurigo nodularis (of Hyde) (Fig. 12.33).

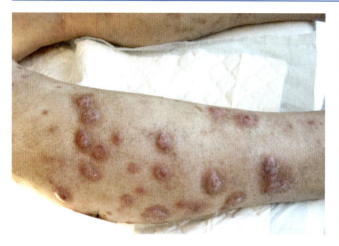

Fig. 12.33

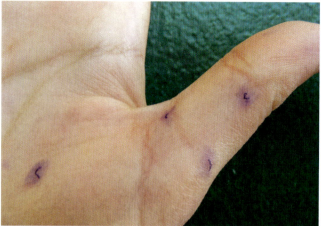

Fig. 12.35

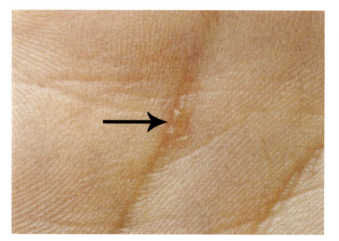

Fig. 12.34

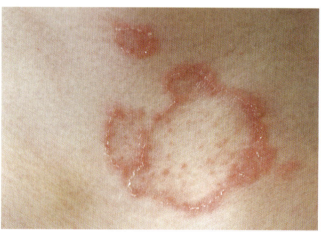

Fig. 12.36

12.10 Scabies

Scabies is a parasitic disease, always endemic, and causing major pruritus in the patient and his or her close contacts (contagiousness). The main findings are signs of scratching (cf. Figs. 12.30, 12.31, and 12.32); anatomic location is often suggestive: anterior axillary lines, genital areas, breasts, hands, wrists, and fingers. The presence of small furrows (cf. Figs. 4.28 and 12.34 (arrow)) must be carefully searched, particularly on the sides of the fingers and the anterior part of the wrists, as they allow confirmation of the diagnosis. In order to make furrows noticeable, they may be colored using a felt pen, then rinsed with water (scabies ink test modified by Frouin); the ink having penetrated inside the furrows remains after rinsing, thus making them apparent (Fig. 12.35).

12.11 Dermatophytosis

Annular lesion with an "active" border, which is elevated and scaly. Circinate dermatophytosis (Fig. 12.36). An annular dermatosis with a scaly border should always be suspected to be a dermatophytosis. In most scaly dermatoses, a mycological examination is desirable because of misleading clinical forms of dermatophytosis which may resemble seborrheic dermatitis (Fig. 12.37) or psoriasis (Fig. 12.38). Clinical appearance is less characteristic in widespread forms treated with topical steroids (*tinea incognita*, Figs. 12.39 and 12.40, note the active border) and in papulopustular variants (Fig. 12.41).

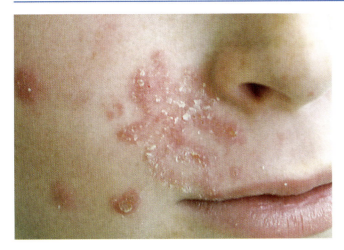

Fig. 12.37

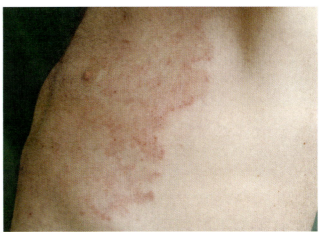

Fig. 12.40

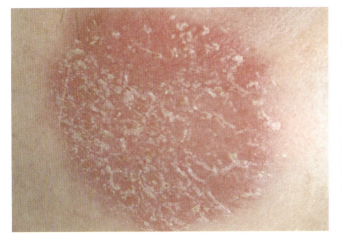

Fig. 12.38

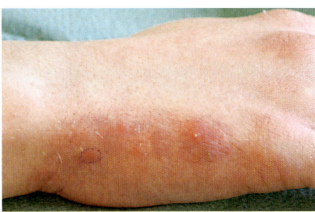

Fig. 12.41

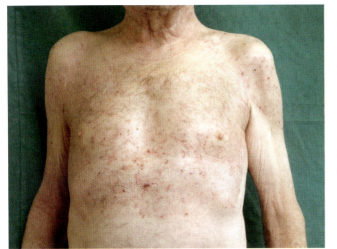

Fig. 12.39

12.12   Impetigo and Ecthyma

Erosive and crusting erythema (Fig. 12.42). Impetigo is a cutaneous infection caused by *Streptococcus* and/or *Staphylococcus aureus*. It is initially bullous, but the bullae are rarely observed since they break quickly and leave an erythema bordered with a collarette (Fig. 12.43); the formation of a honey-colored yellow crust is characteristic (Fig. 12.44; cf. Figs. 2.8 and 7.17). Folds and periorificial areas are often affected. Ecthyma is a necrotic impetigo which progresses deeper in the skin and is preferentially located on the legs (Fig. 12.45).

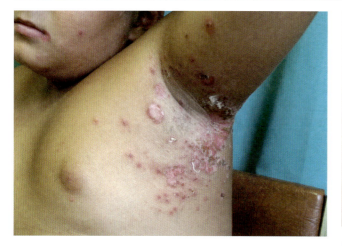

Fig. 12.42

Fig. 12.45

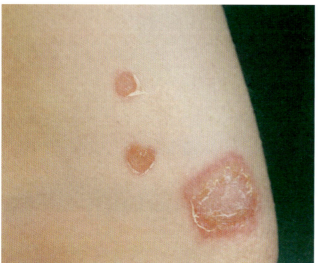

Fig. 12.43

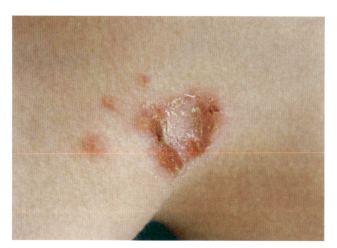

Fig. 12.44

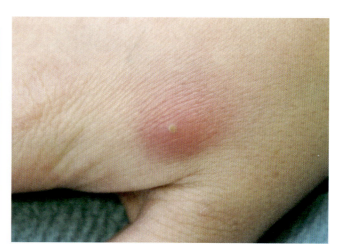

Fig. 12.46

12.13 Pyodermas

Inflammatory nodule. Furuncle (Fig. 12.46). The yellow "boil core" in the center of this nodule is typical of a furuncle, which is one type of pyoderma caused by *Staphylococcus aureus*.

12.14 Acute Soft Tissue Infection (Cellulitis): Erysipela

Erythema (Figs. 12.47 and 12.48). Three signs allow the diagnosis of erysipela: the *sudden* appearance of an *erythematous macule or plaque* in a patient with *fever*. Erysipela of the face is characterized by a sharp peripheral demarcation, with raised borders (Fig. 12.47); this type of sharp demarcation hardly manifests on lower limbs (Fig. 12.48).

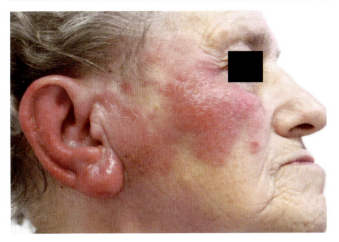

Fig. 12.47

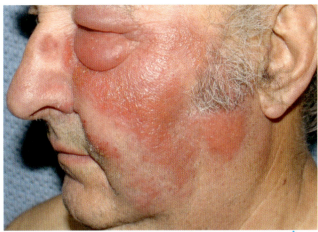

Fig. 12.49

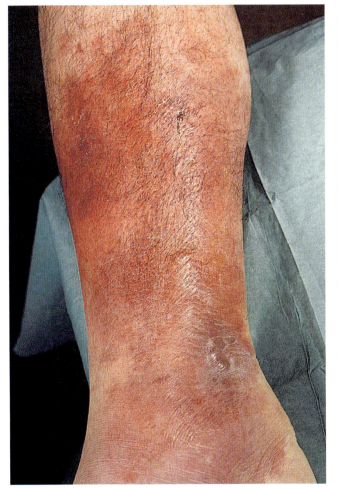

Fig. 12.48

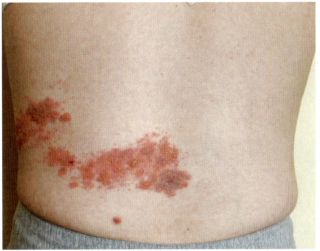

Fig. 12.50

12.15   Herpes, Zoster, and Varicella

Plaques covered with vesicles and bullae (Fig. 12.49) in a dermatomal distribution (V-2). Zoster's primary lesion is an erythema covered with grouped gray vesicles evolving towards umbilication, crusting, and sometimes necrosis, but without oozing. Zoster is caused by a reactivation of the varicella zoster virus. If recognized as such, the segmental (dermatomal) distribution of the lesions imposes the diagnosis (Figs. 12.49 and 12.50). However, it is not obvious on the limbs and scalp. Varicella can easily be identified because of the presence of primary lesions of different stages (vesicle, umbilicated vesicle, crust) (Fig. 12.51 and cf. Fig. 2.11). Herpes is characterized by grouped vesicles/pustules on an erythematous background (Fig. 12.52 and cf. Fig. 1.2). Primary infection is generally more marked than recurrence. Affection of the fingers (herpetic whitlow) can be misleading (Fig. 12.53). The notion of recurrences occurring on a fixed topography is a good argument for diagnosis; isolation of the virus (by PCR or culture) enables a sure diagnosis.

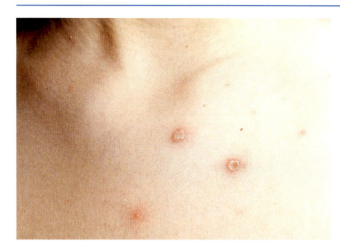

Fig. 12.51

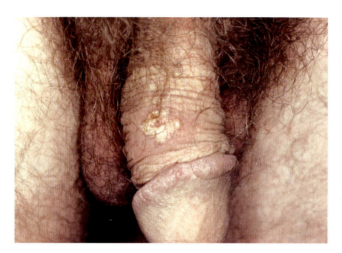

Fig. 12.52

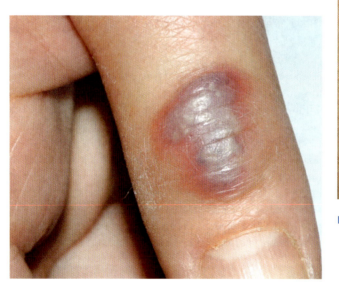

Fig. 12.53

12.16 Warts and Molluscum Contagiosum

Multiple white-gray papules. Molluscum contagiosum (Figs. 12.54 and 12.55). These lesions are smooth, firm, and hemispherical; they are often multiple in children. Umbilication is characteristic (cf. Fig. 4.3), but not always present, as in this example. There are several clinical forms of warts including plantar "mosaic" warts (Fig. 12.56), flat warts (Fig. 12.57), and palmar warts (Fig. 12.58). A profusion of warts can be one of the signs of immune deficiency.

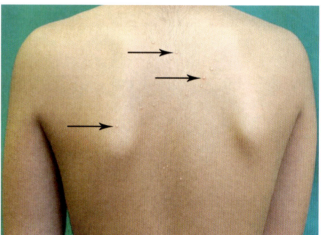

Fig. 12.54

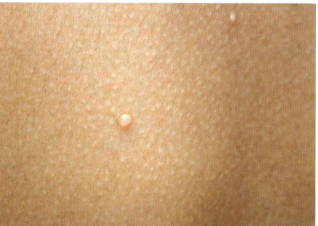

Fig. 12.55

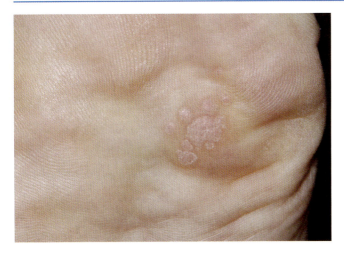

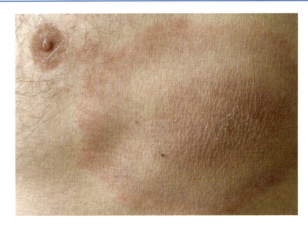

Fig. 12.59

Fig. 12.56

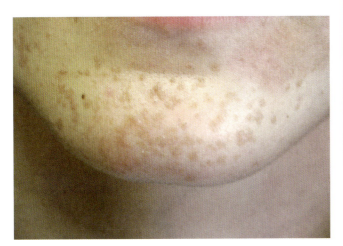

Fig. 12.57

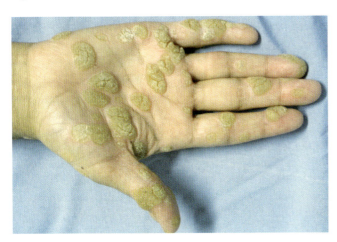

Fig. 12.58

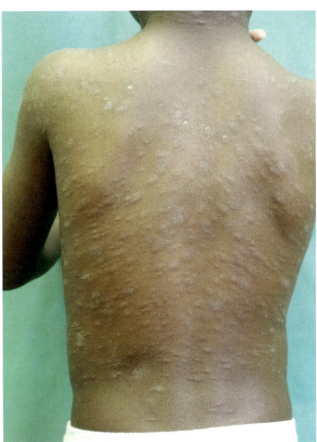

Fig. 12.60

12.17   Other Infections

Centrifugal annular erythema. Erythema migrans. Lyme borreliosis (Fig. 12.59). The red middle part corresponds to the tick bite. However, it is the concentric peripheral ring which migrates slowly (around 0.5 cm/day) in Europe that is characteristic of this disorder. Diagnosis is based exclusively on clinical evaluation and commands an antibiotic treatment with cyclines or amoxicillin, in order to avoid extracutaneous complications of the disease (particularly neurological, cardiac, and articular).

Exanthema. Pityriasis rosea Gibert (Fig. 12.60). It is one of the most frequent and benign exanthemas. It has the

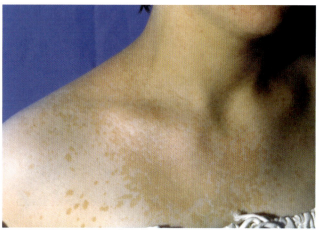

Fig. 12.61

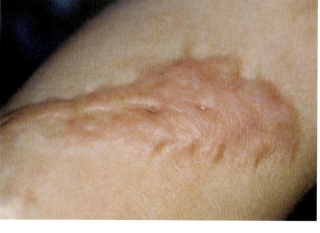

Fig. 12.62

particular feature of being a long-lasting exanthema (4–6 weeks). The most typical form is illustrated here but there are numerous semiological variants. Note:

- The primary lesion, which is a red, scaly macule, papule, or dry plaque (difficult to observe on dark skin)
- The type of scaling: a collarette, i.e., a circular scaling which is loose in the center and adherent in the periphery
- The "pine tree" distribution on the trunk

The rash often appears several days after the preceding initial lesion, known as heraldic (i.e., "which announces").

Confluent buff brown macules. Pityriasis versicolor (Fig. 12.61). The primary lesion is a buff brown or erythematous macule with a fine scale that can evolve towards depigmentation.

12.18 Scar

Flesh-colored plaque, slightly erythematous. Cheloid (Fig. 12.62). Note the lateral extensions in a "crab-leg" pattern, characteristic of cheloid scars. They are permanent and unsightly. This appearance is different from that of simple hypertrophic scars which end up flattening (cf. Fig. 4.28).

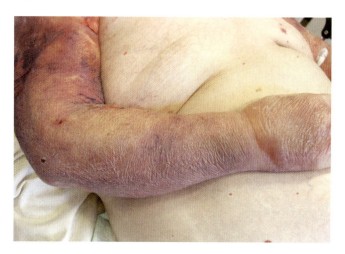

Fig. 12.63

12.19 Dermatoporosis: Skin Aging (Senile Skin)

Fine, wrinkled and ecchymotic, atrophic skin (Fig. 12.63). This appearance is typical of dermatoporosis, which is a chronic cutaneous insufficiency. The skin is fine, transparent in some areas and dark brown in others, covered with linear or stellar scars (Fig. 12.64), and displaying ecchymotic purpura. This type of skin is extremely fragile. The simple act of moving these patients can cause extensive skin collapse, since the skin comes off in large flaps in response to

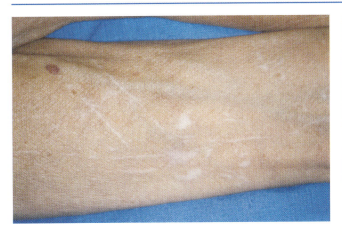

Fig. 12.64

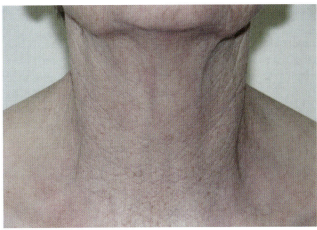

Fig. 12.66

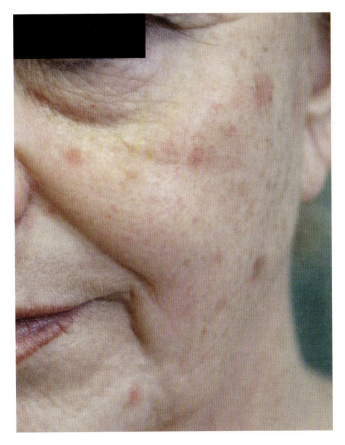

Fig. 12.65

the slightest trauma. The cutaneous signs of photoinduced aging are well visible on Fig. 12.65 and include brown spots (lentigo), wrinkled and atrophic skin, telangiectasias, and the yellow appearance of the inferior eyelid, related to a photo-triggered degradation of the elastic fibers (solar elastosis). The light yellow or lemonlike skin of the anterior neck, showed on Fig. 12.66, is also a sign of skin aging.

12.20 Ulcers: Trophic Disorders

Phlebectases and varicosities. Chronic venous insufficiency (Fig. 12.67). These multiple dilated venules become apparent in the context of venous insufficiency. Venous ulcer (Fig. 12.68, cf. Fig. 7.8) is typically located around the medial malleolus. Also note the other signs of venous insufficiency on Fig. 12.68: phlebectases, pigmentary changes of venous insufficiency (ochre dermatitis), and edema. Arteritis has been illustrated in Fig. 14.17. Figure 12.69 illustrates an ulceration of neurological (neurotrophic) cause. It is a plantar keratotic plaque with central ulceration. The disease should be explored using a buttoned cannula to assess depth of the ulceration and whether it reaches the bone. This type of ulceration is always the consequence of a marked reduction in sensitivity related to a neuropathy, of which it is a late sign. Also note the deformation of the foot, which is large and flat, almost cubical. This is another consequence of the neuropathy.

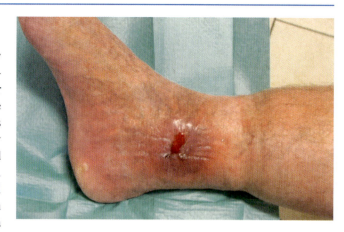

Fig. 12.68

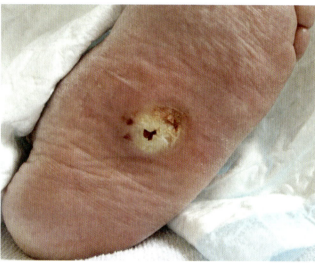

Fig. 12.69

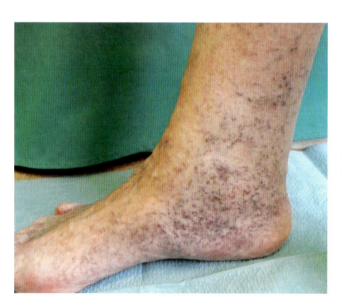

Fig. 12.67

Tumors and Tumorlike Lesions

Most individuals reaching adulthood are likely to develop a cutaneous tumor during their lifetime. Most of these tumors are benign. Some of them are malignant, either because of their ability to grow indefinitely and to invade local tissues, thus causing death (e.g., basal cell carcinoma), or because of their metastatic ability to spread (e.g., melanoma). For teaching purposes, this chapter presents certain lesions which are not tumors in the strict sense, but can suggest the possibility of this diagnosis (e.g., stucco keratosis, venous lake).

13.1   Tumors and Benign Proliferations

13.1.1 Seborrheic Keratosis

Papules and brown keratotic plaques (Fig. 13.1). Seborrheic keratosis is a very common benign tumor, particularly in patients over 60 years old. Most seborrheic keratoses are pigmented, which calls for differential diagnosis with nevi and melanomas. Since this type of tumor is so common, every physician should be able to recognize it, at least in its typical form. It is a proliferation of epidermal cells with characteristic clinical appearances such as papules, plaques, or nodules that are generally keratotic, with sharp demarcations and rectangular borders (lesion appears as if laid on the skin), roughness on palpation, horny plugs (intralesional keratoses that originate from dilated ostia of hair follicles), and color ranging from light brown to dark brown, and are sometimes heterochromatic (Fig. 13.2). In Castellani's disease, numerous brown keratotic papules similar to those found in seborrheic keratosis can be observed on dark skin, in the facio-cervical areas and the upper trunk (also called dermatosis papulosa nigra, Fig. 13.3). When seborrheic keratoses are eruptive, multiple, and inflammatory, they can be the manifestation of a paraneoplastic syndrome (Leser-Trélat sign).

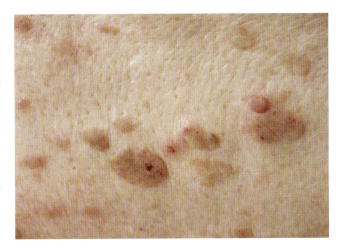

Fig. 13.1

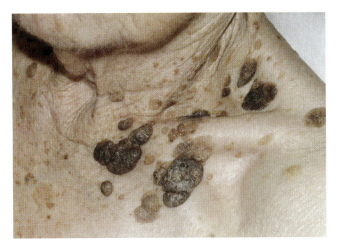

Fig. 13.2

D. Lipsker, *Clinical Examination and Differential Diagnosis of Skin Lesions*, DOI 10.1007/978-2-8178-0411-8_13, © Springer-Verlag France 2013

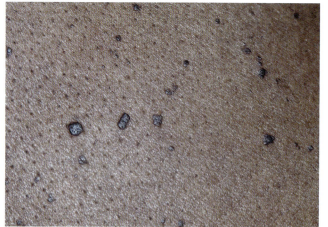

Fig. 13.3

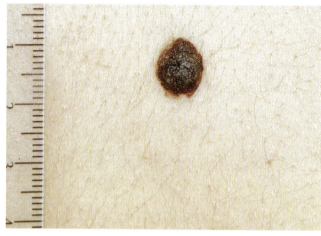

Fig. 13.5

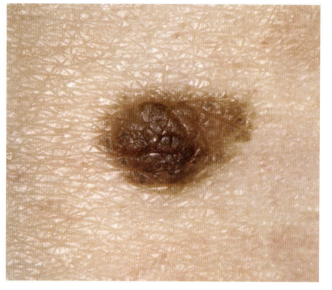

Fig. 13.4

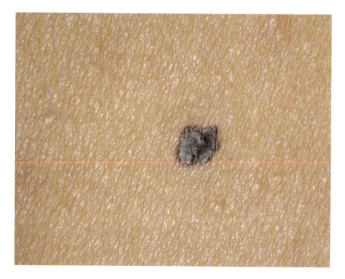

Fig. 13.6

13.1.2 Nevus

Hemispheric, brown, and dome-shaped papule of slightly less than 1 cm wide (Fig. 13.4). A nevus is commonly referred to as a mole. This type of tumor is very common on white skin (Fig. 13.5). It can be a macule, a papule, or a nodule. The size and shape are variable (Fig. 13.6). Color ranges from light brown to black; there are also bluish variants (Fig. 13.7) and even achromic nevi. The surface may be multilobulated (or mammillate) (Fig. 13.4). A nevus can be acquired or congenital. Congenital lesions are often large (Fig. 13.8). A white ring may surround one or more nevi (Sutton's phenomenon or Sutton's nevi); some of these nevi will thus involute and become achromic (Fig. 13.9). The occurrence of a Sutton's phenomenon commands a thorough examination, since it may be synchronous to an evolving

Fig. 13.7

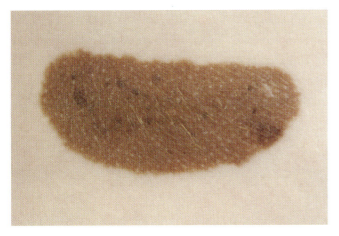

Fig. 13.8

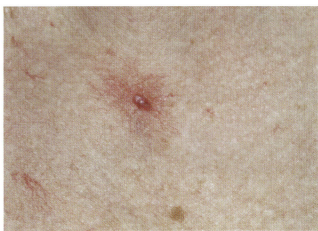

Fig. 13.10

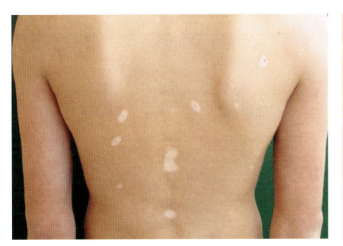

Fig. 13.9

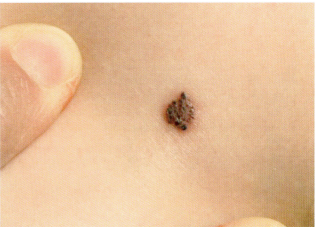

Fig. 13.11

melanoma. When several nevi are affected (Sutton's disease, Fig. 13.9), it can also be a forewarning sign of vitiligo.

Characteristics such as symmetry, evenness, and absence of evolutivity allow distinguishing a nevus from a melanoma.

13.1.3 Vascular Lesions

Red telangiectatic spot with an angiomatous papule in its center. Spider nevus (or nevus araneus) (Fig. 13.10). Pressure exerted on the central papule "empties" the lesion, which reappears by centripetal filling, after pressure is taken off. This type of angioma is quite common; it can appear during pregnancy and disappear after delivery. Multiple spider nevi may indicate a state of relative hyperestrogenism and be one of the cutaneous signs of hepatic cirrhosis.

Reddish-black papule. Thrombosed angioma (Fig. 13.11). Note the peripheral, blue-black, and even spots. This type of lesion is sometimes clinically mistaken for a melanoma.

However, anamnesis will find the notion that there has been a preceding red lesion which has changed rapidly over a few days and become painful. A biopsy is indispensable in case of doubt.

Fleshy and erosive nodule, partially covered with epidermis (epidermalized), that complicates an ingrown nail (Fig. 13.12). Botryomycoma (also known as pyogenic granuloma or proud flesh). Proud flesh (Fig. 13.13) usually occurs rapidly. These lesions may resemble achromic melanoma, especially when located in extremities (cf. Fig. 13.29).

Bluish papule. Venous lake (Fig. 13.14 (arrow)). This lesion is depressible on palpation and can be emptied, which confirms its vascular nature. These lesions are also often located on lips.

Angiomatous papules of variable size (1 mm–1 cm). Ruby spots (or dots, or cherry angioma) (Fig. 13.15). Most of the time, they are in fact palpable lesions. These lesions are smooth, relatively firm on palpation, and of characteristic ruby-red color.

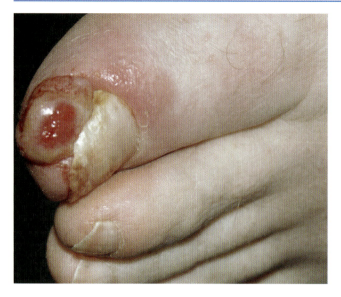

Fig. 13.12

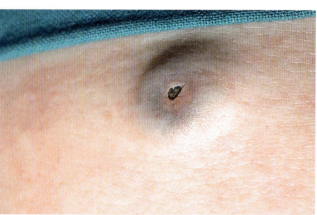

Fig. 13.15

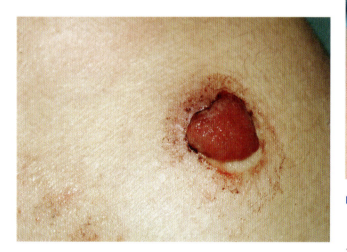

Fig. 13.13

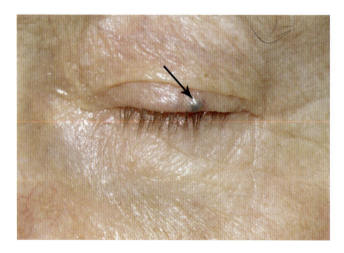

Fig. 13.14

Fig. 13.16

13.1.4 Cysts

Nodule with a central opening. Epidermoid (or infundibular) cyst (Fig. 13.16). This type of cyst is very common. It can lead to aseptic inflammatory flares (Fig. 13.17), in which case the cyst has the appearance of a furuncle (cf. Fig. 12.45). Milia are very small epidermoid cysts (Fig. 13.18). Scalp cysts ("loupe" in French) are very similar but are the result of a different keratinization process; from a histopathological point of view, they are pilar (or trichilemmal) cysts. These cysts are different from real sebaceous cysts, which can be observed in sebocystomatosis (Fig. 13.19). When puncturing a sebaceous cyst, the material is easily extracted and is not foul-smelling, unlike with epidermoid or pilar cysts. Such material can be either filamentous or oily.

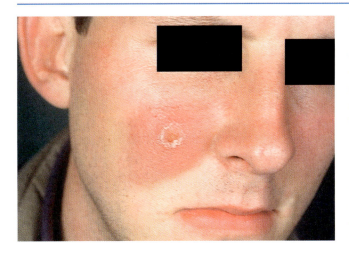

Fig. 13.17

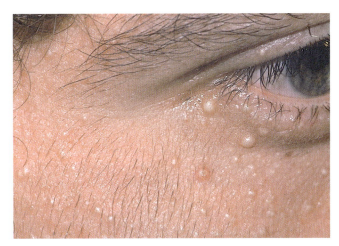

Fig. 13.18

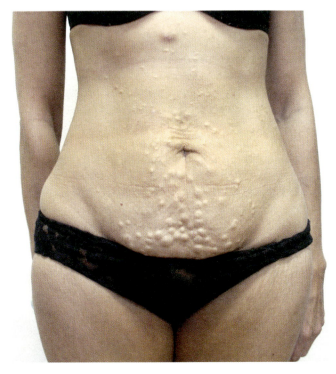

Fig. 13.19

13.1.5 Other Lesions

Gray-white keratotic papules (keratosis). Stucco keratoses (Fig. 13.20, arrows). Stucco keratoses are mostly located on feet and legs. They have a rough appearance and can be easily detached using a curette. This process may cause slight bleeding. These lesions are benign.

Flesh-colored to yellow-white papules with a central depression or dell. Sebaceous hyperplasia (Fig. 13.21, arrows). Also note the telangiectasias. These lesions can sometimes be mistaken for sclerodermiform basal cell carcinoma, desmoplastic trichoepithelioma, and microcystic adnexal carcinoma/syringomatous carcinoma, thus requiring a biopsy. They occur frequently in patients treated with calcineurin inhibitors such as cyclosporin.

Multiple soft nodules, without alteration of the cutaneous surface. Multiple lipomas (Roch-Leri mesosomatous lipomatosis, Fig. 13.22). Lipomas are mobile relative to the deeper-seated musculoaponeurotic system. They are mostly isolated but can be multiple in certain particular contexts (i.e., Roch-Leri mesosomatous lipomatosis, Cowden syndrome, Bannayan-Riley-Ruvalcaba syndrome). The author

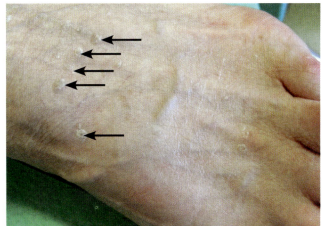

Fig. 13.20

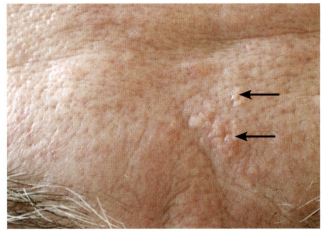

Fig. 13.21

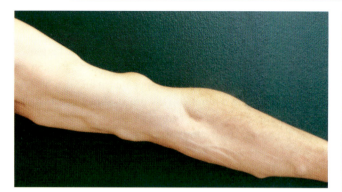

Fig. 13.22

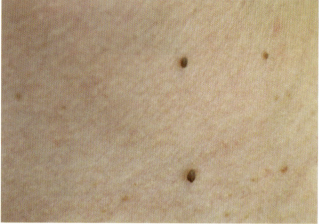

Fig. 13.24

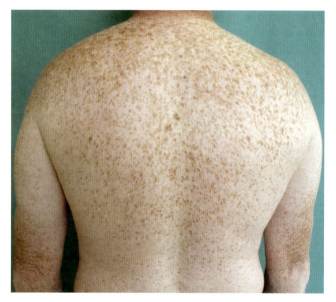

Fig. 13.23

of this book has seen several patients with multiple lipomas (mesosomatous lipomatosis) and melanomas.

Pigmented, brown macules located on the back leading to a "mottled back" appearance. "Flaques solaires," in the French terminology or "sunburn freckles" (Fig. 13.23). These confluent lesions of varying size and shape are typical of "sunburn freckles." They occur after sunburn. They thus allow the diagnosis of a history of previous sunburns, even though the patient would no more remember them.

Soft exophytic papules. Acrochordon or skin tag (Fig. 13.24). Skin tags are very common benign excrescences, located mainly in cervical and inguinal areas. If they are multiple in young patients, they can indicate insulin resistance.

13.2   Malignant Tumors and Cancer

Only the three main cutaneous cancers will be discussed.

13.2.1 Melanoma

Heterochromatic and uneven plaque (Fig. 13.25). Melanoma is the most serious skin cancer. There is no effective treatment of advanced forms. Cure is only achieved with early diagnosis and excision. It is therefore important not to overlook these tumors, which is one of the major challenges of dermatological examination.

The ABCDE rule has been set up to enable large-scale detection of melanoma by a population that has not been specifically trained for this task. Hence, any *asymmetrical* lesion, with irregular *borders*, different *colors*, and a *diameter* of more than 6 mm and which is *evolving*, i.e., is changing (regardless of the parameter taken into account), is suspected to be a melanoma. However, numerous nevi are wrongly suspected to be melanomas, and conversely, numerous melanomas, particularly those evolving rapidly, do not conform to the ABCD criteria.

There are numerous clinical forms of melanomas, only some of which are illustrated here. Most often, it is a macule, a plaque, or a brown, heterochromatic nodule, uneven and asymmetrical (Figs. 13.25 and 13.26). Yet melanoma can be symmetrical (Fig. 13.27) and relatively homogeneous (Fig. 13.28) with little or no pigmentation (Figs. 13.29, 13.30, and 13.31), hence the need to excise all lesions that cannot be diagnosed clinically or with dermatoscopy.

Plantar melanomas, which are frequently covered with a thick keratosis (Fig. 13.32), are particularly difficult to diagnose and easily mistaken for a wart (cf. Fig. 12.55) or a cutaneous horn (cf. Fig. 7.1).

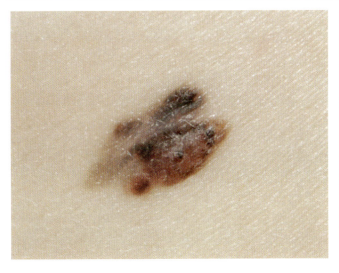

Fig. 13.25

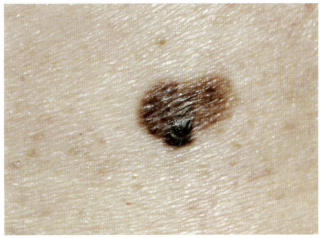

Fig. 13.28

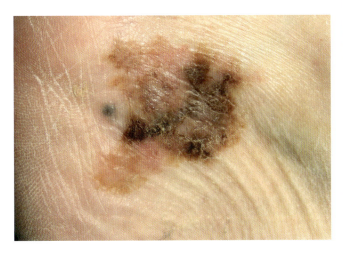

Fig. 13.26

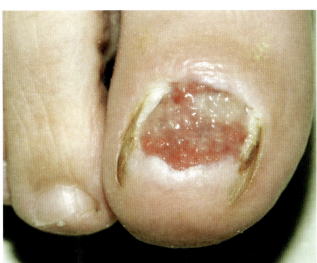

Fig. 13.29

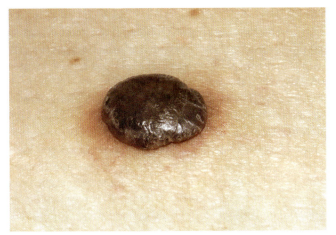

Fig. 13.27

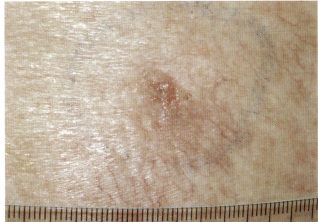

Fig. 13.30

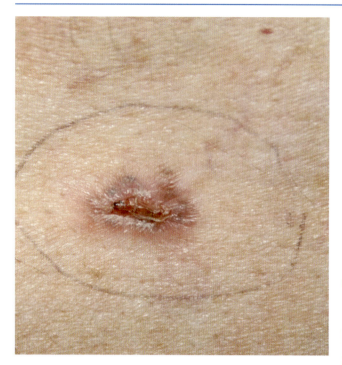

Fig. 13.31

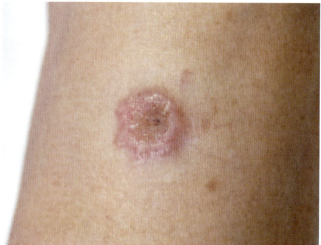

Fig. 13.33

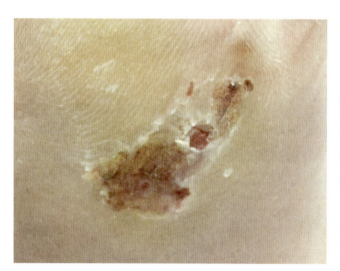

Fig. 13.32

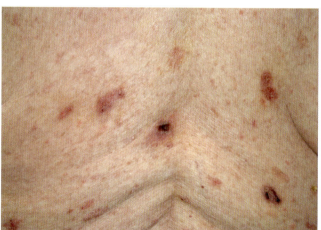

Fig. 13.34

13.2.2 Basal Cell Carcinoma

Translucent, telangiectatic nodule, with a central ulceration. *Ulcerating nodular basal cell carcinoma* (Fig. 13.33). Basal cell carcinoma is the most frequent human cancer, after actinic keratosis (a type of superficial squamous cell carcinoma). There are several clinicopathological variants: superficial with macules and erythema-tous plaques which are more or less scaly and/or keratotic (Fig. 13.34), nodular (Fig. 13.35), terebrant and ulcerative (noduloulcerative), and sclerodermiform (morpheiform); lesions can be pigmented (Fig. 13.35) and may evolve towards central scarring (Fig. 13.36) or ulceration (Fig. 13.33). The most typical aspect which allows clinical diagnosis is the "pearl" (Figs. 13.35 and 13.37). It is a smooth, translucent, gray lesion (papule or nodule), crossed by fine telangiectasias. The whole basal cell carcinoma can be a pearl, especially in nodular forms (Fig. 13.37); sometimes small pearls must be searched on the borders of the lesion (Fig. 13.36). Most basal cell carcinomas are located on the head and the neck. Superficial forms are mostly located on the trunk.

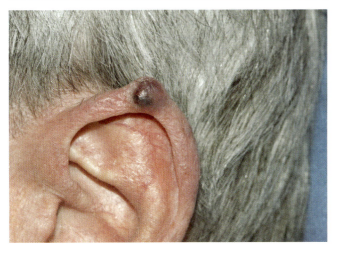

Fig. 13.35

13.2.3 Spinous Cell Carcinoma

Retroauricular ulcer (Fig. 13.38). There are superficial forms of squamous cell carcinoma as well as deep forms, also known as invasive. Most authors consider actinic keratosis (Fig. 13.39, arrows) or Bowen's disease (Figs. 13.40 and 13.41) to be "precancerous" or in situ lesions, whereas histopathologically, they are superficial forms of squamous cell carcinoma. Erythroplasia (of Queyrat) is a mucosal equivalent of squamous cell carcinoma (Fig. 13.42). Superficial forms appear as macules, papules, or scaly and/or keratotic erythematous plaques (Figs. 13.39, 13.40, and 13.41); deeper forms appear as papules, nodules, or tumors which are keratotic (especially the variant known as keratoacanthoma, Fig. 13.43) or ulcerated (cf. Fig. 4.19) and more or less lobu-

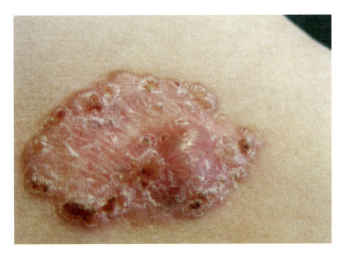

Fig. 13.36

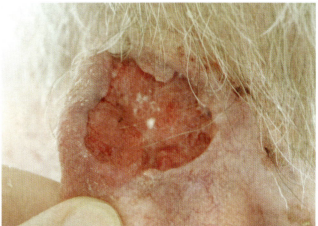

Fig. 13.38

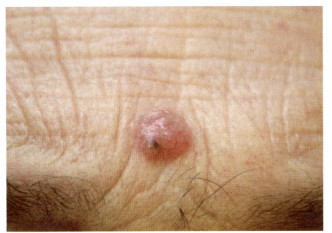

Fig. 13.37

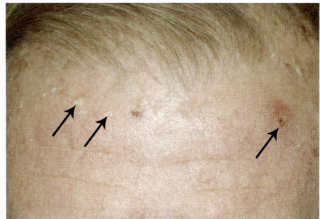

Fig. 13.39

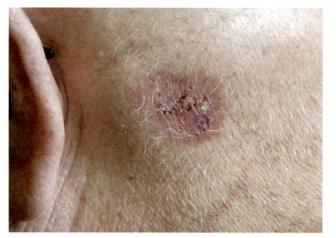

Fig. 13.40

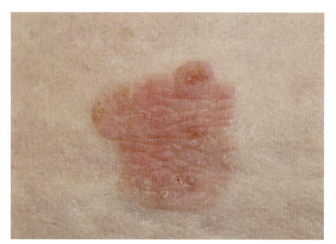

Fig. 13.41

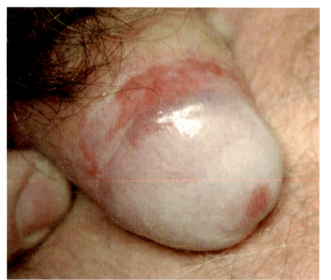

Fig. 13.42

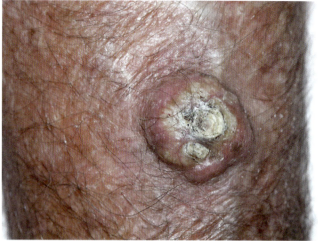

Fig. 13.43

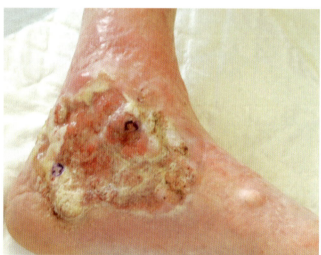

Fig. 13.44

lar and ulcerated (Fig. 13.44), or even terebrant ulcers (Fig. 13.38). Similarly to basal cell carcinoma, squamous cell carcinoma is mainly located on the head and neck. However, other locations are not exceptional since any chronic inflammatory dermatosis and any chronic wound can give rise to a spinous cell carcinoma; Fig. 13.44 illustrates a squamous cell carcinoma of the malleolar area, as a consequence of long-standing inflammation resulting from a chronic graft-versus-host reaction.

Dermatological Signs of Medical Emergencies

14

It would be impossible to cover all cutaneous manifestations of medical emergencies. Here are some important signs indicating diseases that can be life threatening.

14.1 Exanthemas and Erythematous Macules

Historically, the term exanthema was used to describe cutaneous lesions that occur in certain infectious diseases. Today, it is used to describe eruptive cutaneous lesions covering the whole integument or part of it. Enanthema is the mucous affection that may be associated to exanthema.

Kawasaki disease. Exanthema which is predominant in the bathing suit area (Fig. 14.1, case of Pr Boralevi, Bordeaux). Even though rare, this disease must always be considered when diagnosing a child with exanthema, especially between 1 and 5 years old (and regardless of the type of rash) (Fig. 14.2). Indeed, the prognosis of Kawasaki disease depends on early diagnosis and treatment with intravenous immunoglobulins and aspirin. If left untreated, up to 25 % of children develop serious aneurysmal cardiovascular complications. The criteria for diagnosis are high persistent fever (>5 days), conjunctivitis (Fig. 14.3), oropharyngeal involvement (cheilitis, saburral tongue which becomes depapillated and "strawberry-like"), edema of the extremities that is more or less erythematous (Fig. 14.4) (followed by characteristic periungual peeling of the skin in large scales, "en doigts de gant" in the French terminology), exanthema, and enlarged cervical lymph nodes. The location of the rash on the buttocks is characteristic (Fig. 14.1); however, the exanthema can be generalized, maculopapular (Fig. 14.2), diffuse and erythematous, or urticarial. BCG reactivation is classical (Fig. 14.5). The general condition is almost always strongly affected.

Monomorphic papular exanthema; certain lesions displaying a darker center (Fig. 14.6). Chronic meningococcemia (case of Dr Cuny, in Nancy). Certain septicemias are chronic and may appear as an exanthema, such as in this example of type B chronic meningococcemia (Fig. 14.6); they may however become devastating. Hence the dogma of performing blood cultures in every patient with a febrile exanthema, especially when recurrent and associated to joint and/or tendon pain or to deterioration of the general condition.

Hardly visible erythematous macule located on the palms (Fig. 14.7, arrow). Janeway lesion (infectious endocarditis). This sign is subtle and evanescent (<48 h), but very specific of subacute infectious endocarditis; in this case, the infection was caused by *Streptococcus oralis*, and it occurred after dental surgery. In endocarditis, palmar erythematous macules sometimes coexist with purpuric lesions (arrow) (Figs. 14.8 and 14.9). There is a continuum between the classic Janeway lesion (Fig. 14.7) and Osler's nodes (cf. Fig. 14.12). The identification of these lesions can be lifesaving as it allows diagnosis of infectious endocarditis.

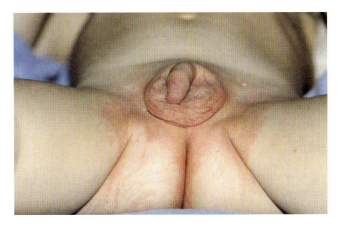

Fig. 14.1 (Photos Courtesy of Pr Boralevi, Dermatology Department, University Hospital of Bordeaux)

D. Lipsker, *Clinical Examination and Differential Diagnosis of Skin Lesions*, DOI 10.1007/978-2-8178-0411-8_14, © Springer-Verlag France 2013

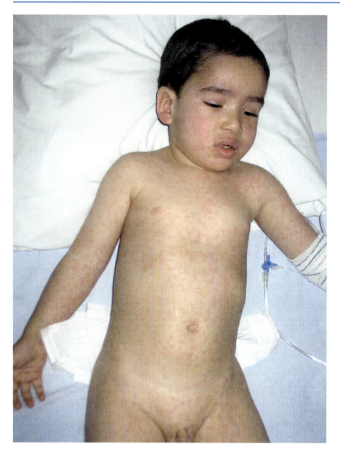

Fig. 14.2   (Photos Courtesy of Pr Boralevi, Dermatology Department, University Hospital of Bordeaux)

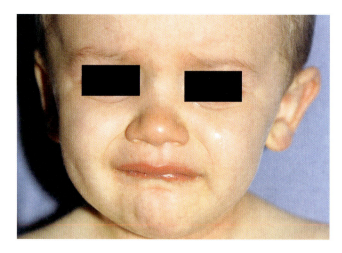

Fig. 14.3   (Photos Courtesy of Pr Boralevi, Dermatology Department, University Hospital of Bordeaux)

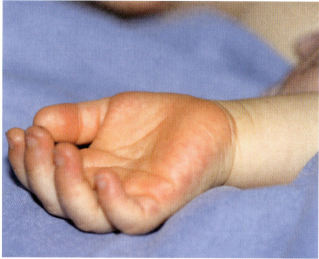

Fig. 14.4   (Photos Courtesy of Pr Boralevi, Dermatology Department, University Hospital of Bordeaux)

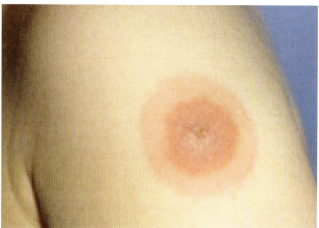

Fig. 14.5   (Photos Courtesy of Pr Boralevi, Dermatology Department, University Hospital of Bordeaux)

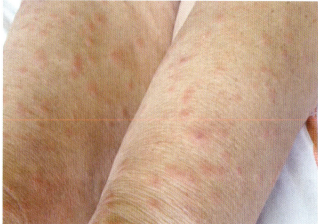

Fig. 14.6 (Photos Courtesy of Dr Cuny, Dermatology Department, University Hospital of Nancy)

14.2 Purpura, Purpura Fulminans, and Livedo. Necrosis

103

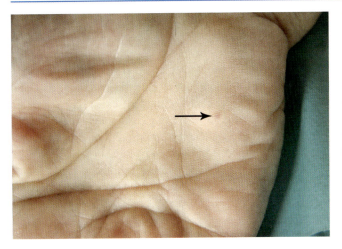

Fig. 14.7

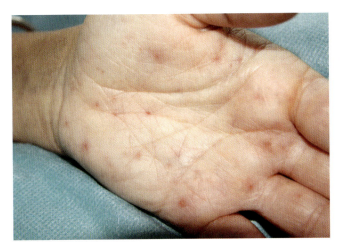

Fig. 14.8

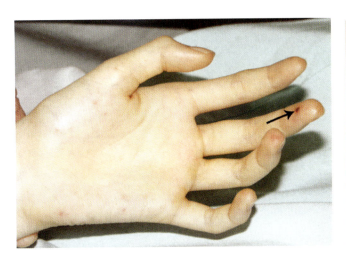

Fig. 14.9

14.2 Purpura, Purpura Fulminans, and Livedo. Necrosis

Acral petechiae (Figs. 14.10 and 14.11). Staphylococcal septicemia. In patients with fever, this type of acral petechiae must suggest a septicemia and/or an endocarditis.

Purpuric macules and papules located on the soles (Osler's nodes, Fig. 14.12). Infectious endocarditis. These lesions can be painful. Their presence imposes blood cultures and ultrasounds (transthoracic and/or transesophageal), even in the absence of fever.

Purpura fulminans (ecchymotic and gangrenous purpura) in disseminated intravascular coagulation (DIC) (Fig. 14.13). Type C meningococcemia (photo Dr Astruc). The main characteristic of this type of purpura is its appearance, which can be reticulate (retiform purpura) and/or stellate and/or maplike. This type of purpura always reflects a thrombosing vasculopathy. The most initial lesions are uneven, purpuric macules. The distinctive characteristic of retiform ("netlike") purpura is its "fullness" (cf. Fig. 14.14): spaces in between

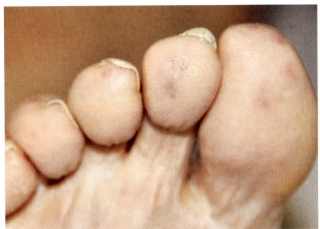

Fig. 14.10

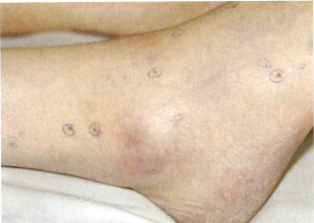

Fig. 14.11

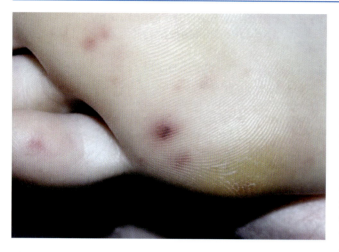

Fig. 14.12

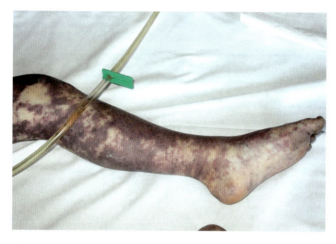

Fig. 14.13 (Photo Courtesy of Dr Astruc, Pediatric Department, Regional University Hospital of Strasbourg)

the meshes caused by purpura are in fact ecchymotic, whereas in common livedo, these spaces have a normal skin color. This type of purpura reveals a disseminated intravascular coagulation (DIC) which can be either tissular or systemic. Therefore, an infectious cause must be searched, first and foremost, although noninfectious diseases can also be responsible for this disorder (e.g., calciphylaxis, homozygous protein C or S deficiency, catastrophic antiphospholipid syndrome, thrombotic thrombocytopenic purpura).

Abdominal and plantar purpura fulminans (Figs. 14.14 and 14.15) with reticulate appearance. Septicemia caused by infection with *Capnocytophaga canimorsus*. This unusual transparency of the soles, where veins are visible, is typical but late developing. The anatomy of the superficial cutaneous venous network can be observed in vivo due to the thrombosis of the entire vascular network, which becomes apparent.

Stellate, map-like purpura. Acute lower limb ischemia (Fig. 14.16). Stellate purpura is a sign always revealing a serious disorder and indicating cutaneous ischemia.

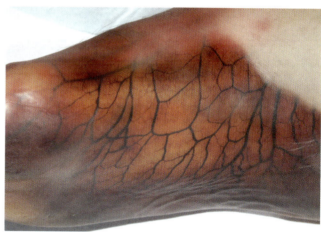

Fig. 14.15

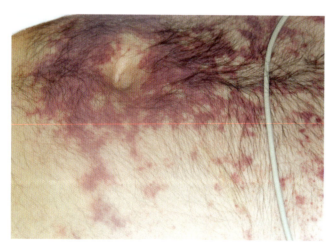

Fig. 14.14

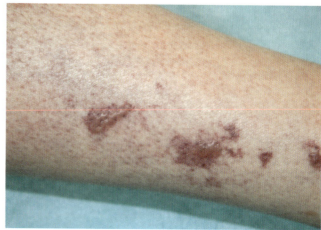

Fig. 14.16

Necrotic detachment of the nail (Fig. 14.17). Critical ischemia. Arteritis. The painful separation of one or several nails of the feet or hands is often the first sign of advanced arteritis, which commands urgent general checkup and treatment. Multiple causes exist: advanced atheromatosis or occlusive arterial disease, Buerger's disease, embolism, hypereosinophilic syndrome, systemic vasculitis, etc.

Hemorrhagic bullae, purpura (Fig. 14.18). This type of hemorrhagic bullae may reflect a coagulopathy (bleeding disorder). It can also be the superficial sign of a necrotizing, deep hematoma which should be dealt with rapidly in order to avoid a devastating necrotic evolution (Fig. 14.19).

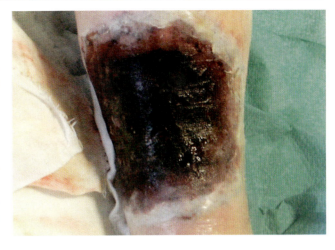

Fig. 14.19

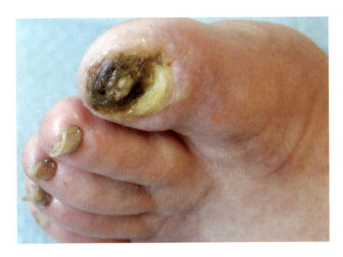

Fig. 14.17

14.3 Pustules

Pustule (arrow) on a purpuric background (Fig. 14.20). Infectious endocarditis. When facing this type of lesion, septicemia must always be suspected. In case of periarticular lesions associated with tenosynovitis, septicemia caused by infection with gonococci must be mentioned and blood cultures performed, as well as sampling of the potential sites of the primary infection (urethra, cervix, anus, pharynx). Similar lesions can be observed in certain autoinflammatory diseases such as Behçet's disease, as well as in other infections (cf. Fig. 12.53).

Pustular eryhtema (Fig. 14.21). Acute generalized exanthematous pustulosis (AGEP). The clinical picture can be spectacular, violent, and febrile and therefore often mistaken for an infection. This is a cutaneous drug reaction that can become complicated by a severe capillary leak syndrome. Generally, erythema starts in the large skin folds (intergluteal, axillary, etc.), where it is predominant, and is secondarily covered with pustules that are sometimes very transient.

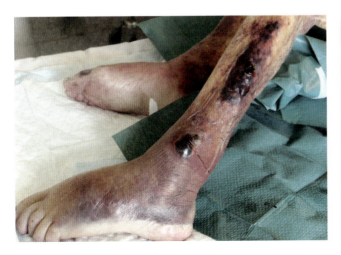

Fig. 14.18

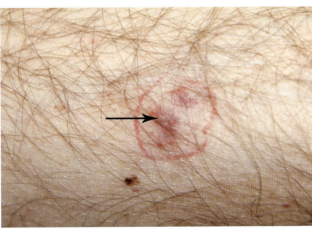

Fig. 14.20

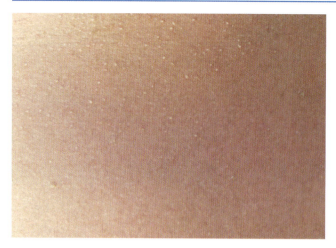

Fig. 14.21

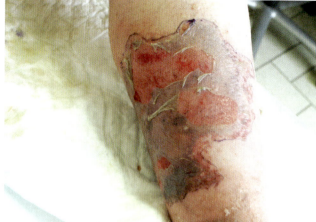

Fig. 14.22

14.4 Bullae and Skin Detachment

Purpura, bulla, skin detachment, toneless, and pale skin (Figs. 14.22 and 14.23). Acute infectious cellulitis (soft tissue infection) of necrotizing evolution. Certain local signs indicate a severe, necrotic evolution of infectious cellulitis; such signs must be searched systematically since these affections present medical and surgical emergencies. The skin is toneless and pale, with erythema presenting irregular borders. A stellate or map-like purpura is present at the periphery and sensitivity is decreased. In the latter case, the insensitive area should be pricked using a needle. This process should normally induce pain. In case of insensitivity (without any pre-existing neuropathy), the situation is extremely severe. Most often, there is no bleeding when the needle is pulled out. These types of soft tissue infection require urgent surgery.

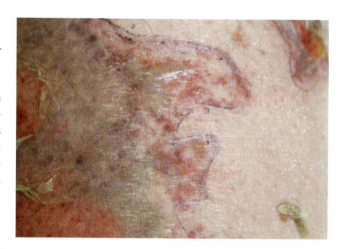

Fig. 14.23

Scalded skin (Figs. 14.24 and 14.25, arrows). Staphylococcal epidermolysis (SSSS = staphylococcal scalded skin syndrome), in a localized and benign variant. This disease is mediated by exfoliatin, a staphylococcal toxin that provokes intraepidermal cleavage, which explains the superficial skin separation. The staphylococcal source must therefore always be searched (particularly omphalitis in newborns and impetigo in older children). An antistaphylococcal antibiotic treatment must also be initiated. In this example, the child had an impetigo caused by infection with a staphylococcus which secretes exfoliatin. He also had distant epidermolysis, at its least severe.

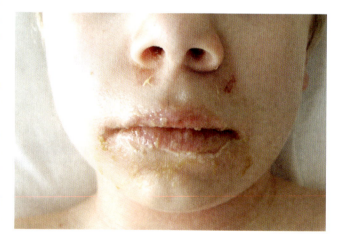

Fig. 14.24

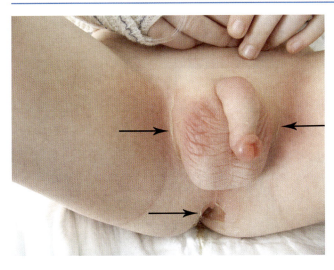

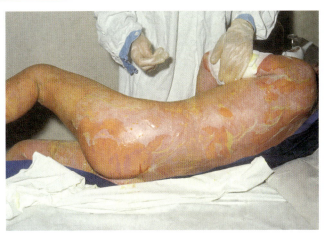

Fig. 14.27

Fig. 14.25

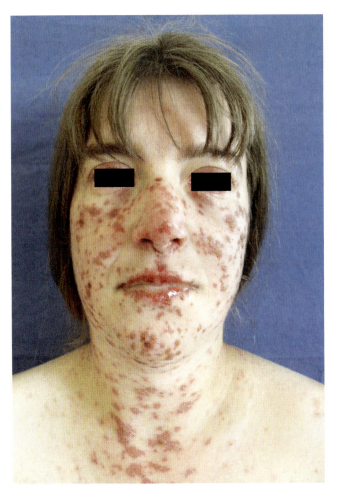

Fig. 14.26

Multiple, erosive, erythematous macules with cheilitis (Fig. 14.26). Stevens-Johnson and Lyell's syndrome. This appearance of the face is typical of the syndrome, which is a severe cutaneous drug reaction that can cause a lethal acute cutaneous failure through extensive skin separation (Fig. 14.27), in a patient with Lyell's syndrome. Lesions often start in the mid face area, as in this patient. The primary lesion is an erythematous macule which evolves into skin separation. Nikolsky's sign can be positive at this early stage (cf. Fig. 8.3). It is imperative to withdraw the drugs that are causing this affection. In case of widespread lesions, most authors recommend treatment with intravenous immunoglobulins.

14.5   Other Signs and Syndromes

Erythroderma (Figs. 14.28 and 14.29). Erythroderma is a generalized erythema, affecting more than 80 % of the cutaneous surface. It is chronic (>15 days, unlike generalized erythema) and rapidly evolves towards scaling. This syndrome has many causes and can be life threatening through associated skin failure. The latter can be responsible for thermoregulation problems, water and protein loss (including anticoagulant C protein, and this is associated with a risk of thrombosis), and a defective skin barrier resulting in high vulnerability to infections.

(Sudden) swelling of the lips. Urticaria of deeper layers of the skin (angioedema, Fig. 14.30). Angioedema can be life

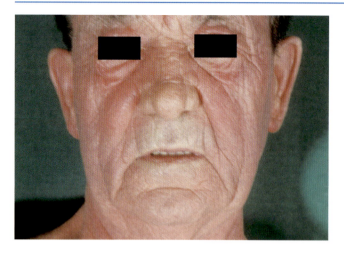

Fig. 14.28

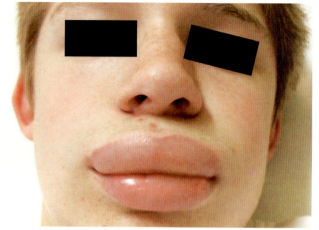

Fig. 14.30

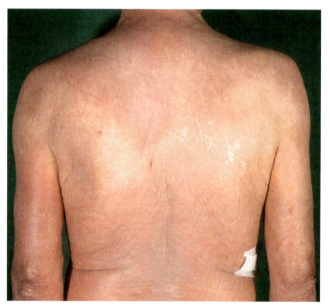

Fig. 14.29

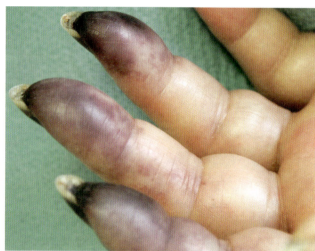

Fig. 14.31

threatening due to constrictive laryngopharyngeal affection. It can also be associated with an anaphylactic shock. It has multiple causes, particularly genetic and drug related.

Acral purpuric cyanosis (acral cyanosis, Fig. 14.31). It often indicates a DIC or a severe affection of the microcirculation and therefore imposes the search for sepsis, blood disorders, and/or thrombotic microangiopathy.

Cutaneous Manifestations of Internal Diseases

15

15.1 Systemic Inflammatory Diseases

15.1.1 Behçet's Disease

Genital aphthosis. Behçet's disease (Fig. 15.1). Mouth and genital ulcers ("bipolar aphthosis"), as well as pustules on an erythematous (Fig. 15.2) and/or purpuric background, are the most suggestive cutaneous signs of this systemic autoinflammatory disease. It particularly involves a risk of thrombophlebitis, aneurysms, uveitis, and inflammation of the central nervous system. Superficial thrombophlebitis (Fig. 15.3) is also more frequent in this disorder. The thrombosed vein can be localized on palpation.

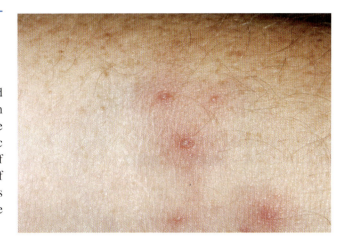

Fig. 15.2

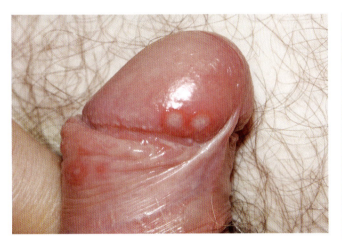

Fig. 15.1

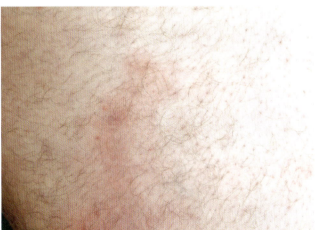

Fig. 15.3

D. Lipsker, *Clinical Examination and Differential Diagnosis of Skin Lesions*, DOI 10.1007/978-2-8178-0411-8_15, © Springer-Verlag France 2013

15.1.2 Lupus Erythematosus (LE)

Malar rash (vespertilio erythema or "butterfly rash"). Acute cutaneous lupus erythematosus in a patient with systemic lupus erythematosus (Fig. 15.4). Cutaneous signs are common in this connective tissue disease which affects nearly all organs, particularly the joints, kidneys, serous membranes, heart, and central nervous system. Some cutaneous signs known as "specific lesions" allow diagnosing the disorder in the absence of other signs of the disease. Indeed, there is a particular histopathological aspect, namely, an interface dermatitis. The complex terminology of these cutaneous signs is a practitioner's concern; only their specificity is of real importance. Other signs allow identifying a subgroup of patients particularly prone to thromboembolic and vascular complications. The main specific lesions are the malar rash (Fig. 15.4), psoriasiform (Fig. 15.5) and/or annular (Fig. 15.6) lesions of subacute cutaneous lupus erythematosus, and lesions of chronic lupus erythematosus (Fig. 15.7). The primary lesion in acute LE is a congestive erythema (Fig. 15.4) that can become scaly. In the course of acute lupus erythematosus, exanthema can be generalized (Fig. 15.8); the presence of lesions on extremities is common (Fig. 15.9). Periungual hyperaemia is a common sign (Fig. 15.10), particularly in infants. In subacute LE, the primary lesion is an erythema of leukodermic evolution, which is gray-white and telangiectatic (Fig. 15.6) and which can be psoriasiform (Fig. 15.5) and/or blistering and crusting, mainly on the borders (periphery) (Fig. 15.11). The following primary signs are associated with chronic LE: erythema, keratosis, dyschromia, and cutaneous atrophy (Fig. 15.7).

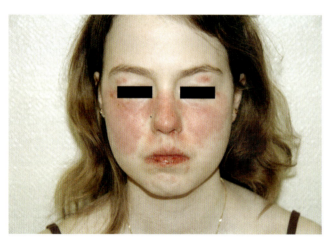

Fig. 15.4

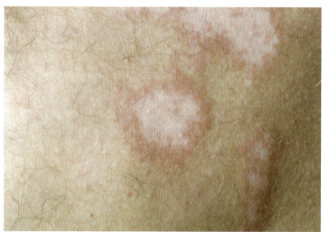

Fig. 15.6

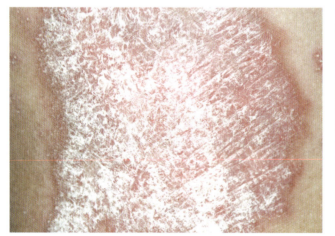

Fig. 15.5

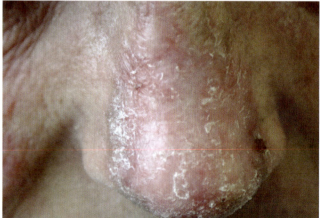

Fig. 15.7

The following lesions occur mainly in patients with systemic lupus erythematosus who are prone to thrombosis: livedo racemosa with non-infiltrated and large meshes (Fig. 15.12) or, conversely, acral fine livedo (Fig. 15.13), livedo vasculitis (Fig. 15.14), depressed porcelain-white papules as encountered in malignant atrophic papulosis or Degos disease (Fig. 15.15), non-infiltrated acral purpura (Fig. 15.16), and anetoderma (cf. Fig. 6.12).

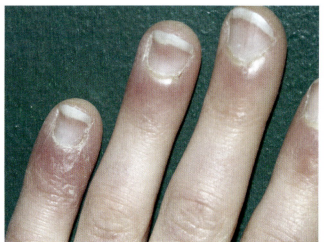

Fig. 15.10

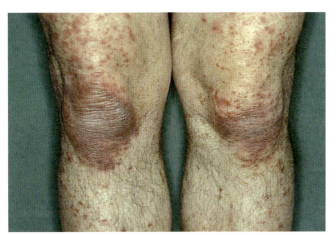

Fig. 15.8

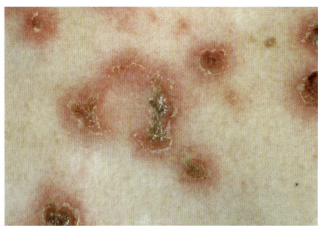

Fig. 15.11

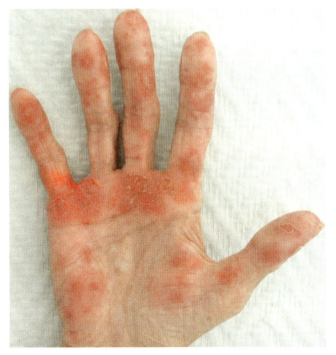

Fig. 15.9

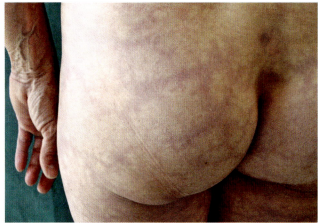

Fig. 15.12

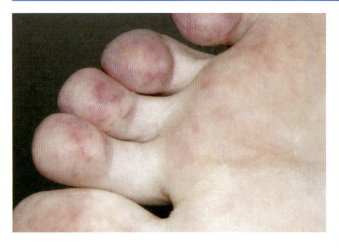

Fig. 15.13

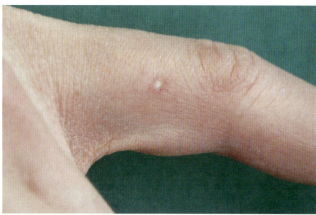

Fig. 15.15

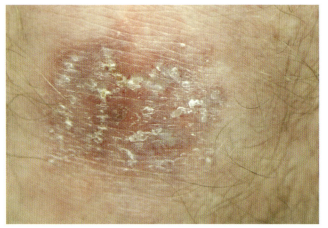

Fig. 15.14

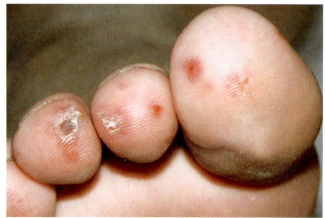

Fig. 15.16

15.1.3 Dermatomyositis

Erythema around the joint surfaces of the back of the hands, particularly the metacarpophalangeal and proximal interphalangeal joints (Fig. 15.17). The cutaneous signs are extremely characteristic of this disorder and allow establishing diagnosis. These signs consist of an erythema which can be papular (Gottron's papules) and is located above the metacarpophalangeal (Fig. 15.18) and proximal interphalangeal joints; these lesions may evolve towards crusting necroses (Fig. 15.19). They can also consist of a linear erythema of the back of the hands (cf. Fig. 1.1) or a flagellate erythema of the trunk (cf. Fig. 9.23), or also an erythema with a very peculiar violaceous coloration, evolving into poikiloderma on the knees, elbows, and/or eyelids (Fig. 15.20). The presence of mega-capillaries (submillimeter-sized telangiectasias) surrounding the nails is common (Fig. 15.21, arrows); a similar appearance can be observed in scleroderma.

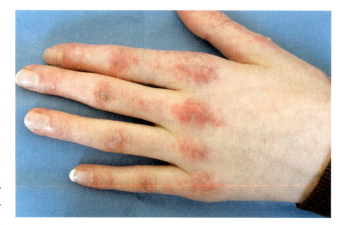

Fig. 15.17

Semiological features in favor of this diagnosis are the violaceous color of the lesions, the presence of telangiectases, and the evolution into poikiloderma. Early diagnosis of dermato-

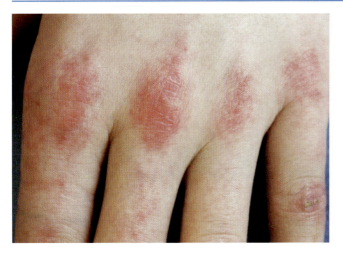

Fig. 15.18

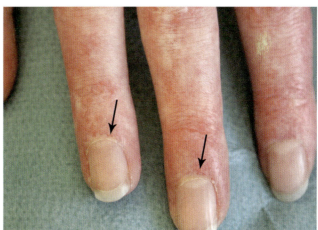

Fig. 15.20

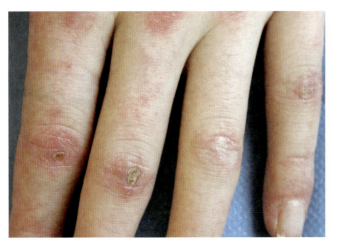

Fig. 15.19

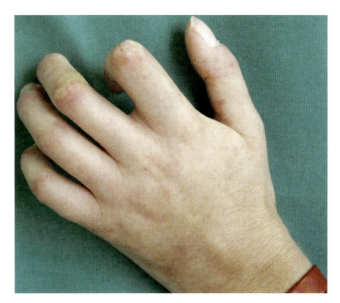

Fig. 15.21

myositis is important since this disorder exhibits several patterns of progression that are severe, including major muscle involvement (swallowing muscles, diaphragm, heart, etc.), a very severe interstitial lung disease, a risk of opportunistic infections (e.g., pneumocystosis), and associated cancer in approximately 15 % of cases.

15.1.4 Systemic Sclerosis

Sclerosis of the hand accompanied by the complete disappearance of skin folds on fingers, as well as retracted fingers (Fig. 15.22). Systemic sclerosis is of complex pathogenesis and unknown cause. Several clinical forms exist and are characterized by a more or less diffuse hardening of the skin, which loses its suppleness (sclerosis). This situation is extremely crippling. The affection is predominant in

Fig. 15.22

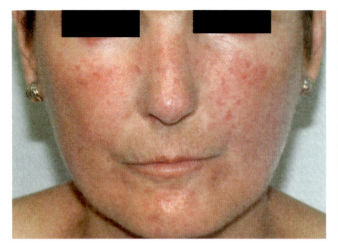

Fig. 15.23

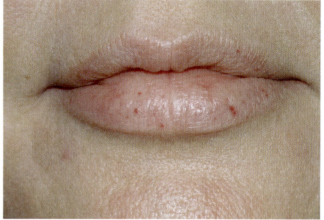

Fig. 15.26

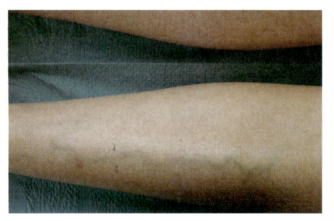

Fig. 15.24

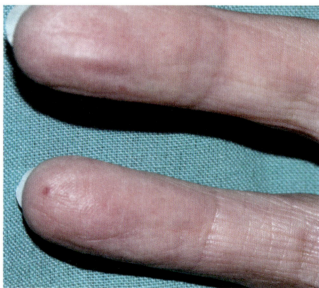

Fig. 15.27

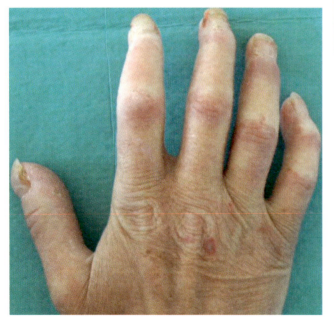

Fig. 15.25

extremities, and fingers end up retracting (Fig. 15.22); the face appears fixed (wrinkles have disappeared except around the mouth (Fig. 15.23)) and is covered with telangiectases. The groove sign is characteristic (Fig. 15.24). Patients with scleroderma almost always present with a Raynaud's phenomenon (Fig. 15.25). They often develop digital ulcers. The presence of rectangular telangiectases on the face (Fig. 15.26) and fingers (Fig. 15.27) is typical. The last phalange must be carefully examined: mega-capillaries are present and there is periungual paleness and sometimes necrosis of the cuticles (Fig. 15.28); fusion of the nail plate with the periungual skin (*pterygium*) is typical (Fig. 15.28). A pigmentation disorder also exists, with a shiny hypopigmentation, particularly visible on pigmented skin (Fig. 15.29).

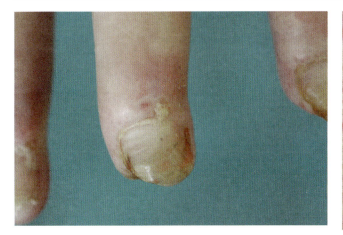

Fig. 15.28

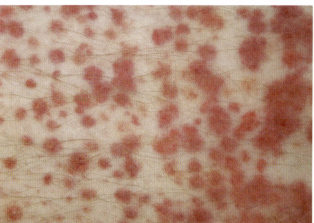

Fig. 15.30

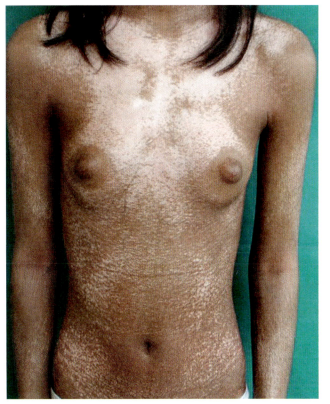

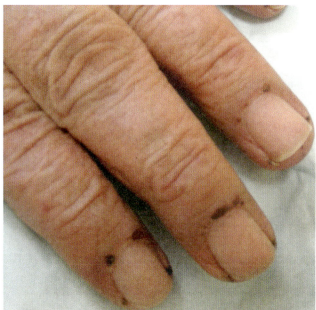

Fig. 15.31

Fig. 15.29

15.1.5 Vasculitis

Palpable purpura. Leukocytoclastic vasculitis (Fig. 15.30). Vasculitis can have several dermatological expressions which are outside the scope of this book. They consist of a group of diseases characterized by an inflammation of the vascular wall, which may cause thrombosis. All organs can be affected and mostly the skin, digestive tract, and kidneys. There are multiple variants of vasculitis, which are classified according to the size of the smallest affected vessel and the presence of certain antibodies (ANCA: anti-neutrophil cytoplasmic antibodies). The most common dermatological expression of all forms of vasculitis is an erythematous and/or purpuric papule (Fig. 15.30). The most common site is the leg, and lesions tend to merge. A necrotic or pustular evolution is possible. Periungual and digital, confluent millimeter-wide purpuric papules are characteristic of rheumatoid vasculitis (Fig. 15.31). An infiltrated livedo accompanied by papules or nodules suggests medium- or large-vessel vasculitis (Fig. 15.32).

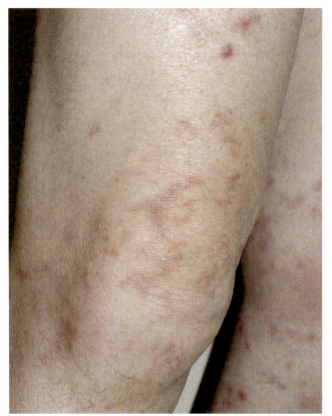

Fig. 15.32

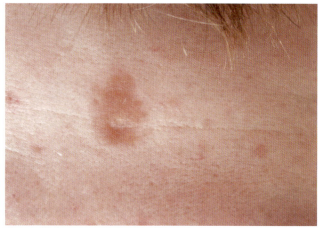

Fig. 15.33

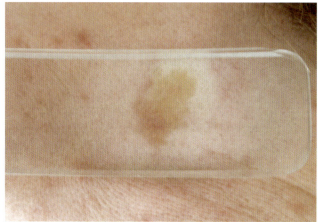

Fig. 15.34

15.1.6 Sarcoidosis

Erythematous plaques which appear lupoid on diascopy (Figs. 15.33 and 15.34). Sarcoidosis is a systemic granulomatous disease of unknown cause. Almost all organs can be affected, particularly the lungs, lymph nodes, eyes, and skin. Cutaneous manifestations are numerous, some of which are not specific, e.g., erythema nodosum (cf. Figs. 5.21 and 5.22). Other specific manifestations are characterized by a granulomatous infiltrate in the dermis and/or hypodermis. In such cases, diagnosis can be established through skin biopsy. The most classic forms are papules (small and large) and plaques. One of the characteristics of these lesions is their lupoid appearance on diascopy. It consists of a yellow coloration which becomes apparent when pressure is exerted on the lesion using a transparent object, which empties the blood contained therein (Figs. 15.33 and 15.34). Lesions are red or red-brown and can be telangiectatic (Figs. 15.35, arrows and 15.36). The affection of the face by erythematous plaques defines the clinical form known as "lupus pernio." The affection of the sides of the nose is known as angiolupoid of Brocq and Pautrier (Fig. 15.36, cf. Fig. 35.7). The cutaneous affection of the nostrils commands the search for

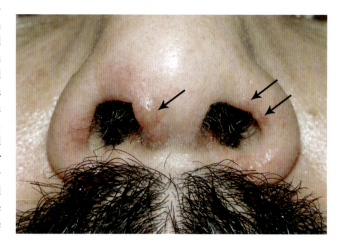

Fig. 15.35

an endonasal affection which can become obstructive and justifies a general treatment. Finally, the infiltration of an old scar (Fig. 15.37) must firstly suggest sarcoidosis; such an

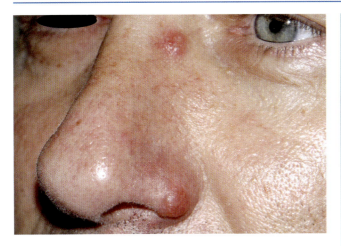

Fig. 15.36

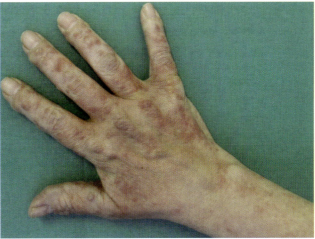

Fig. 15.38

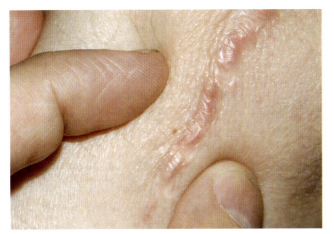

Fig. 15.37

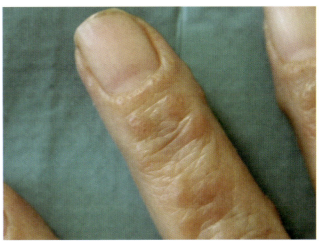

Fig. 15.39

infiltration can also be seen in recurrences of cancer and certain parasitoses (coccidioïdomycosis, sporotrichosis).

15.1.7 Multicentric Reticulohistiocytosis

Multiple, flesh-colored, or erythematous and violaceous papules of the back of the hands (Fig. 15.38). Multicentric reticulohistiocytosis is an arthrocutaneous syndrome causing a destructive symmetric polyarthritis resembling rheumatoid arthritis. The dermatological appearance is quite characteristic: it is a papulonodular rash starting on the dorsa of the hands where it is predominant (Fig. 15.38), especially the proximal nail fold involvement which has a characteristic "coral bead" appearance (Fig. 15.39). These are firm, dermal lesions, without alteration of the cutaneous surface. Biopsy of such lesions allows establishing diagnosis since the histopathological appearance is pathognomonic and reveals a granulomatous infiltrate with multinucleated cells and a ground glass appearance.

15.1.8 Reactive Arthritis and SAPHO Syndrome

Focal keratoderma (keratoderma blennorrhagica) (Fig. 15.40, arrow). Apart from real psoriatic lesions, circinate balanitis, and conjunctivitis, a very peculiar form of keratoderma may occur in patients with reactive arthritis: it is an acquired focal keratoderma with "tack-like" lesions (Fig. 15.40, arrow) that are very rough and keratotic in the center, with a smoother but raised periphery, resembling a tack. "Reiter's syndrome" should not be used to describe this situation since this author was a notorious Nazi who had been directly involved in the slaughter of innocent people. Psoriatic dactylitis is often associated to a yellow thickening of the nail plate, which can also crumble off, as in this figure (Fig. 15.41). Aseptic acral pustulosis of the palms and soles (Fig. 15.42) can be the manifestation of SAPHO syndrome (which combines many of the following features: synovitis, acne, pustulosis, hyperostosis, and osteitis).

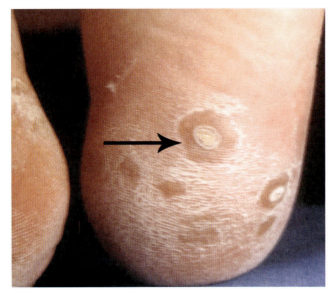

Fig. 15.40

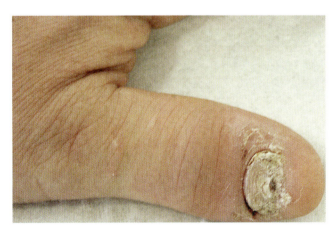

Fig. 15.41

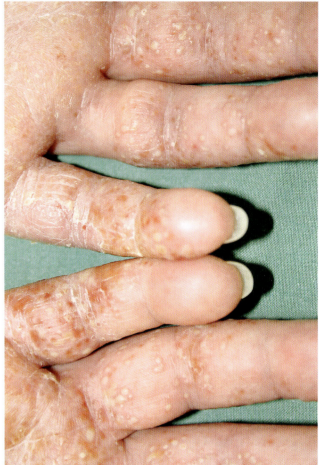

Fig. 15.42

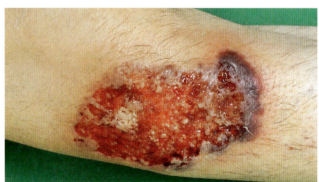

Fig. 15.43

15.1.9 Pyoderma Gangrenosum

Ulcer with a purpuric halo, which appears undermined (Fig. 15.43). Pyoderma gangrenosum belongs to a group of disorders called neutrophilic diseases, because the inflammatory flare-ups are associated with neutrophilic tissue infiltration. Sweet syndrome (cf. Fig. 4.12) and subcorneal pustulosis of Sneddon-Wilkinson are other examples. Affection of the skin is the most common, although most organs can be affected (hepatosplenomegaly, lung disease, osteitis, meningitis, etc.). Pyoderma gangrenosum is a painful and widespread ulceration characterized by a purulent periphery which confers to the border an undermined appearance (Figs. 15.43 and 15.44); the border is erythematous and/or purpuric (Fig. 15.43). The initial primary lesion, which is rarely observed in clinical practice, is a follicular (aseptic) pustule. There may be high fever, which compli-

cates differential diagnosis with an acute infectious cellulitis, as in this example where pyoderma gangrenosum has initially been mistaken for severe erysipela (Fig. 15.45). This disorder is significantly associated with myeloid blood disorders and cryptogenetic inflammatory diseases of the intestine.

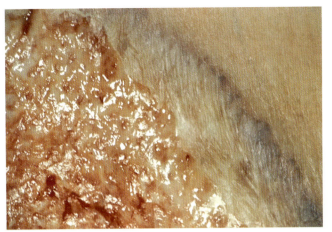

Fig. 15.44

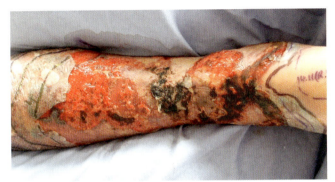

Fig. 15.45

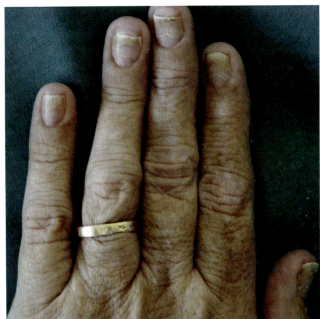

Fig. 15.46

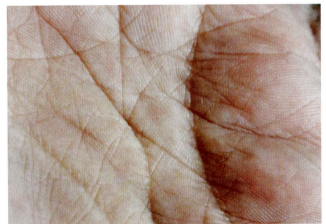

Fig. 15.47

15.1.10 Cronkhite-Canada Syndrome

Pigmentation of the back of the hands associated with distal onycholysis and proximal separation of the nail plate (onychomadesis) (Fig. 15.46). It is a non-hereditary polyposis which rarely turns into cancer and is associated with a severe exudative bowel disease causing diarrhea accompanied by weight loss and edema. This syndrome is currently considered as an inflammatory disease. The cutaneous signs are common and quite characteristic: hyperpigmentation, particularly of the folds and palms (Fig. 15.47). Constant modifications of the appendages are nail appearing yellow and separated (xanthonychia and onycholysis) (Fig. 15.46) and alopecia.

15.1.11 Chilblain

Violaceous papules and plaques of the back of the toes (Fig. 15.48). Chilblains (pernio) are papules and erythematous or violaceous plaques, appearing on the dorsa of the fingers (Fig. 15.49) and toes (Fig. 15.48) and sometimes elsewhere (nose, ear lobules, Achilles tendon, knees), in cold and humid weather. Certain edematous forms of chilblain

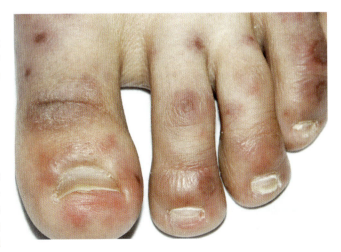

Fig. 15.48

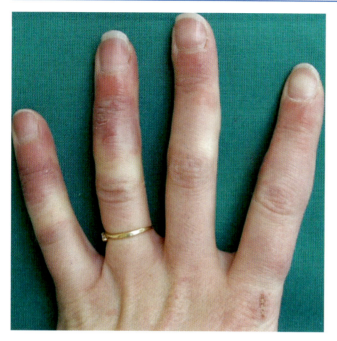

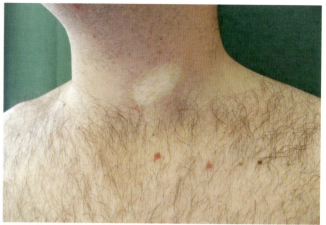

Fig. 15.50

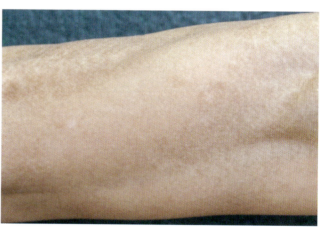

Fig. 15.49

should not be confused with synovitis. They persist for approximately 15 days before disappearing. They are often idiopathic but can be the manifestation of various systemic diseases, including chronic myelomonocytic leukemia, lupus erythematosus, antiphospholipid antibody syndrome, cryo-globulinemia, cryofibrinogenemia, cold agglutinin-induced diseases, and Aicardi-Goutieres syndrome. Chilblains which occur or persist until summer are usually symptomatic of a connective tissue disease.

Fig. 15.51

15.1.12 Morphea

Pearl-white, oval, sclerous plaque occurring in the cervical area (Fig. 15.50). Morphea should not be mislabeled as "localized scleroderma," even though skin biopsy does not allow distinguishing them. Indeed, there is no transition between these two entities. There are several variants of morphea, the most severe forms being the *linear forms* (Figs. 15.51, 15.52, and 15.53), which are mainly found in children. They can cause limb atrophy (Figs. 15.51 and 15.52) and, when located on the face, hemifacial atrophy (Fig. 15.53) as well as anomalies of the central nervous system (epilepsy, learning gaps, etc.). The linear forms are often associated with biological markers of autoimmune conditions such as antinuclear factors and must be treated by experienced practitioners. The *plaque form* morphea are either isolated or multiple scleroatrophic plaques, either pigmented (Fig. 15.54) or white and sclerotic (Fig. 15.50); they are more common and benign forms.

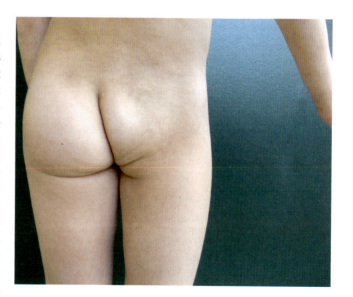

Fig. 15.52

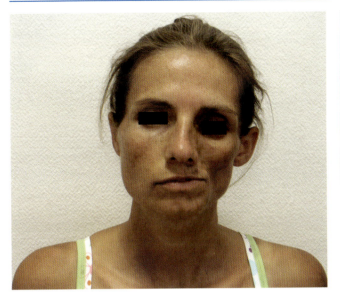

Fig. 15.53

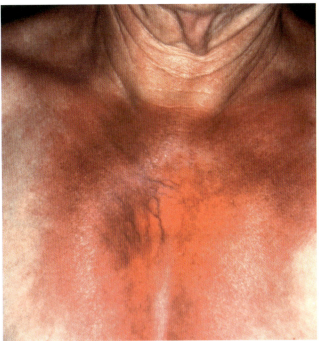

Fig. 15.55

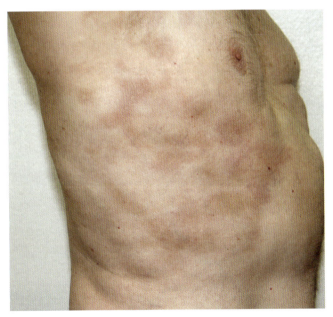

Fig. 15.54

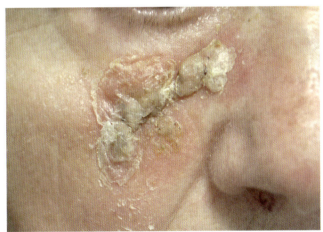

Fig. 15.56

15.1.13   Contiguous Inflammation of the Skin (or Inflammation by Contiguity)

Erythema with blunt but marked borders and exaggerated visibility of the vessels. Contiguous inflammation of the skin in AESOP syndrome (adenopathy and extensive skin lesion overlying plasmacytoma, Fig. 15.55). Inflammation by contiguity is hardly taught and described in reference books, despite its clinical relevancy. It is an erythema that can be associated with an alteration of the cutaneous surface (scales, crusts, Fig. 15.56). This erythema is located above a deep-seated source of inflammation, i.e., an infection or a tumor, which is not directly related to it. Figures 15.55, 15.56, 15.57, and 15.58 illustrate a few examples, i.e., a widespread erythema surrounding a gouty arthritis of the knee that can be easily mistaken for erysipela (Fig. 15.57), a crusting erythema of the face that appeared during flare-ups of sinusitis (Fig. 15.56), a gingival erythema around the source of a dental infection (Fig. 15.58), and an erythema with marked but blunt borders and particularly visible vessels which extends over a solitary plasmocytoma of the sternum (AESOP syndrome, Fig. 15.55).

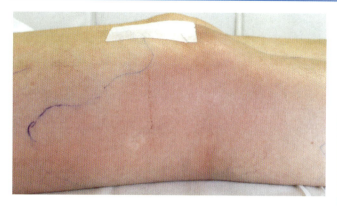

Fig. 15.57

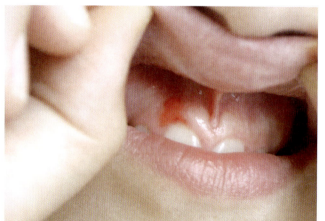

Fig. 15.58

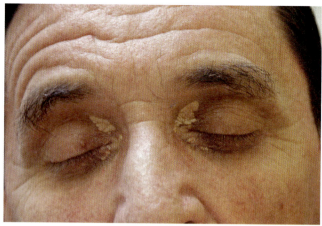

Fig. 15.59

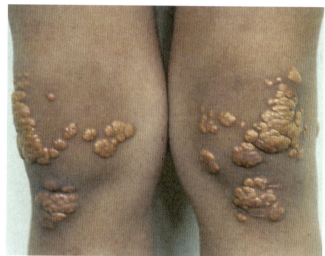

Fig. 15.60

15.2   Endocrinopathies and Nutrition-Related Diseases

15.2.1 Xanthomas

Periorbital yellow papules and plaques. Xanthelasma (Fig. 15.59). The various clinical forms of xanthoma can be diagnosed through skin biopsy, which reveals the presence of xanthoma cells in the dermis (i.e., cells containing an excess load of fats). Clinically, yellow papules and plaques are observed, without alteration of the skin surface (Figs. 15.59 and 15.60). Tuberous xanthomas (Fig. 15.60) are associated with hypercholesterolemia that must be searched. Eruptive xanthomas (cf. Fig. 4.1) are associated with hypertriglyceridemia. Xanthelasmas (Fig. 15.59) are quite common after 40. Before that, hypercholesterolemia and monoclonal gammopathy must be searched; the latter must be looked for in adults regardless of age in case of extensive xanthelasma or widespread xanthoma. Simple xanthelasmas should not be mistaken for necrobiotic xanthogranuloma (Fig. 15.61), which is often associated with myeloma.

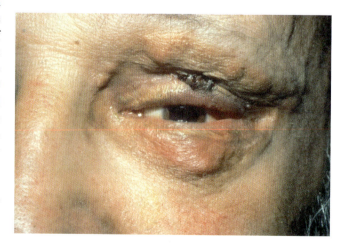

Fig. 15.61

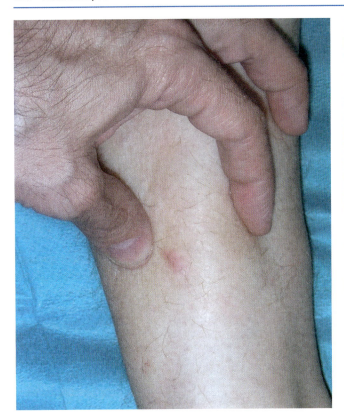

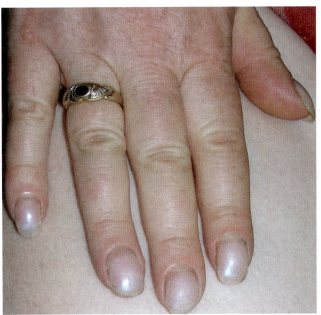

Fig. 15.63

Fig. 15.62

15.2.2 Pretibial Myxedema

Pretibial myxedema is the cutaneous expression of Graves' disease, and it often occurs after surgical treatment of the latter. It is characterized either by a palpable induration while the cutaneous surface appears normal (Fig. 15.62) or by erythematous plaques and nodules that can become confluent. In very rare situations, it can result in elephantiasis. In any case, the pretibial location is typical. The posterior-external aspect of the forearms can be affected, although this is rare. Myxedema is often associated with exophthalmia and thyroidal acropathy (Fig. 15.63), accompanied by clubbing of the fingers and rough nails (as if brushed with sandpaper, i.e., trachyonychia).

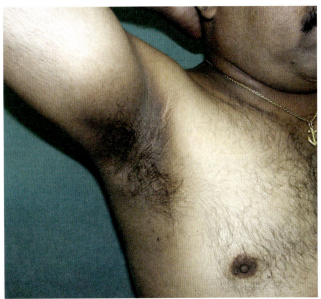

Fig. 15.64

15.2.4 Pellagra

Photodistributed erythema which is accompanied by superficial scaling and which evolves towards pigmentation (Fig. 15.65). It is the result of vitamin PP deficiency which is characterized by a triad of "diarrhea-dementia-dermatitis" that can cause death, if not treated. The dermatitis is a sun-exposed edematous erythema which rapidly turns into diffuse scaling and the formation of a collarette that evolves towards pigmentation. These disorders are very rare nowadays, except in specific circumstances: major undernutrition, alcoholism, anorexia nervosa, and short bowel syndrome, as in Fig. 15.65.

15.2.3 Acanthosis Nigricans

Brown, keratotic, digitated "dirty" appearance of the axillary fold (Fig. 15.64). The "filthy" and rough appearance of the axillary and inguinal folds, in particular, and of the neck is characteristic. Acanthosis nigricans most often indicates insulin resistance and/or diabetes. When it is of recent onset and unusual location (back of the hands, palms, circumoral), it is the marker of a visceral cancer (stomach, lungs, etc.) and behaves like a paraneoplastic syndrome.

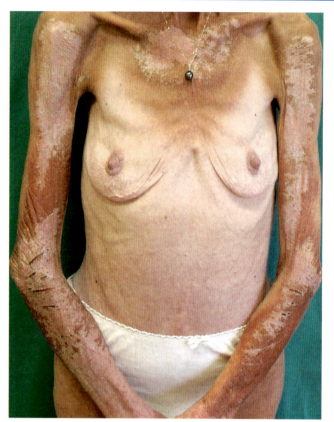

Fig. 15.65

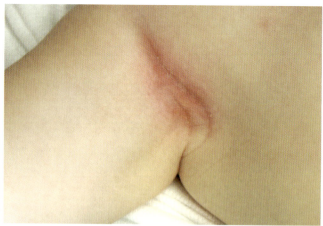

Fig. 15.66

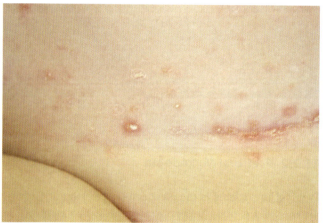

Fig. 15.67

15.3 Cell Proliferative Diseases

15.3.1 Langerhans Cell Histiocytosis

Persistent intertrigo of the newborn (Fig. 15.66). Langerhans cell histiocytosis often includes cutaneous signs. A red or scaly and crusting intertrigo that is resistant to usual treatments (Fig. 15.66). It can be accompanied by red, scaly, or crusting papules located close by or at a distance (Fig. 15.67); these papules may cover the trunk in a characteristic undershirt distribution. Scales are often fatty; collarette scaling is common. Such lesions are also sited on the scalp (Fig. 15.68) and are easily misdiagnosed as "cradle cap" (seborrheic dermatitis of the newborn). Langerhans cell histiocytosis is a proliferative disorder (abnormal proliferation of histiocytes) that is probably reactive. The affections of the bones (swelling, fractures) and of the hypothalamic-pituitary axis (diabetes insipidus) are common.

15.3.2 Mastocytosis

Turgescence of reddish-brown macules on rubbing (Darier's sign, Figs. 15.69 and 15.70). Cutaneous mastocytosis

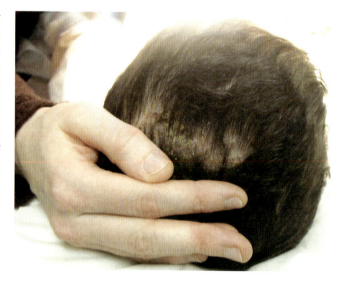

Fig. 15.68

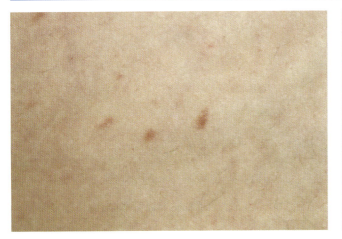

Fig. 15.69

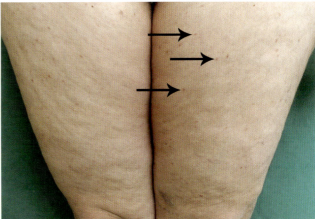

Fig. 15.71

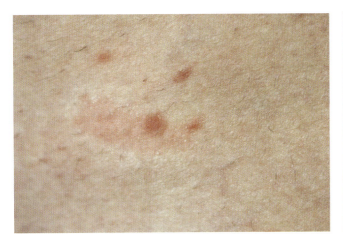

Fig. 15.70

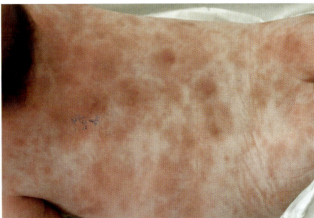

Fig. 15.72

(urticaria pigmentosa type). Involvement of the skin and bones is very common in mastocytosis. The following manifestations are relatively common. Urticaria pigmentosa (Fig. 15.71) consists of brown (arrows) or coppery macules that become turgescent on rubbing (Darier's sign, Figs. 15.69 and 15.70). This sign is of no value in a patient with dermographism (cf. Fig. 12.20). A cutaneous mastocytoma consists of one or several yellow plaques; it is found mainly in infants and can become bullous during baths. In diffuse cutaneous mastocytosis (Fig. 15.72), the skin is infiltrated with erythematous and confluent plaques and nodules. Mastocytoses can involve only the skin (cutaneous mastocytosis) or it can involve different other organ systems (systemic mastocytosis). In the systemic forms, functional impairment of organs must be determined, as it is the most reliable sign of an aggressive variant. The most commonly affected organs are the bones (osteoporosis),

the digestive tract (ulcer, diarrhea), the liver (elevation in transaminase levels), the urinary system (pollakiuria), and the central nervous system (mood disorders and memory problems).

15.4 Paraneoplasias

15.4.1 Ichthyosis

Polygonal scale/keratosis that is relatively adherent. Ichthyosis is a common hereditary disease, characterized by dry and rough skin with more or less polygonal, adherent scales. If an adult patient develops acquired ichthyosis (Fig. 15.73), the search for certain diseases is mandatory, such as sarcoidosis, lupus erythematosus, and thyroid dysfunction; drug intake, i.e., statins; and mostly lymphoma or cancer.

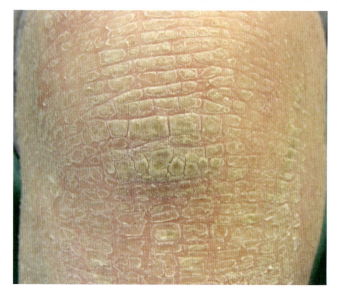

Fig. 15.73

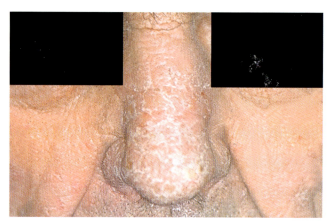

Fig. 15.74

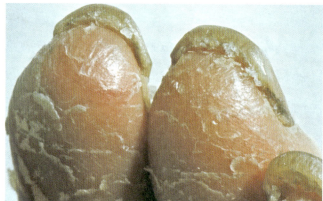

Fig. 15.75

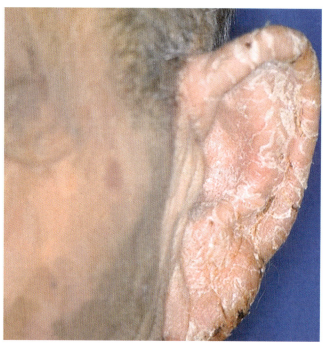

Fig. 15.76

15.4.2 Acrokeratosis Paraneoplastica

Acquired keratosis of the nose (Fig. 15.74). Acrokeratosis paraneoplastica is always a paraneoplastic syndrome. It is most often associated with cancer of the upper aerodigestive tract; cervical adenopathy is generally palpable on diagnosis, since the cancer has already spread. It is an acquired acral keratosis which starts at the fingertips (Fig. 15.75) and quickly spreads to the nails. The latter become yellow (xanthonychia), thick (subungual hyperkeratosis), and detached (onycholysis); the nose bridge and pinna can be affected (Fig. 15.76); the affection resembles psoriasis, for which it is a differential diagnosis. This diagnosis should be suspected in alcoholic and smoking patients in their 50s with a de novo appearing acral "psoriasis." At a later stage, involvement of the fingers, toes, and face becomes more pronounced, with a marked keratosis of the helix and nose bridge, as well as a keratoderma (Fig. 15.77); at this point, the cancer has invariably spread. In its final stage, the affection may be diffuse.

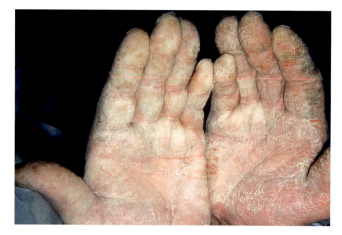

Fig. 15.77

15.5 Susceptibility to Cancers

15.5.1 Cowden Syndrome

Leukokeratosis with a papillomatous pattern of the gums (Fig. 15.78, arrows). This syndrome is a genetic predisposition to breast and thyroid cancers, particularly by mutation of the *PTEN* gene. From the dermatological point of view, it is characterized by the presence on the face of multiple papules, which are usually small and flesh-colored, sometimes very discreet, sometimes digitated like warts, and histologically classified as trichilemmomas (Fig. 15.79, arrows), as well as a papillomatous leukokeratosis of the gums (Fig. 15.78). These patients may also have acral keratoses and multiple lipomas.

15.5.2 Muir-Torre Syndrome

Crusted nodule and multiple flesh-colored papules (on the cheeks and nose). Sebaceous carcinoma and adenoma (Fig. 15.80). Muir-Torre syndrome is a variant of Lynch syndrome, by mutation of the genes involved in the repair of incorrectly paired nucleotides (NER, nucleotide excision repair, i.e., *MSH1*, *MLH2*). These patients develop cancers of the colon, as well as urothelial and endometrial cancers. From a dermatological point of view, they develop papules and/or multiple papulonodules on the face, which are often accompanied by alterations of the cutaneous surface (ulcers, crusts, etc.) corresponding to sebaceous tumors, particularly sebaceous carcinoma and adenoma (Fig. 15.80). If a single sebaceous adenoma or carcinoma is diagnosed, the search for the Muir-Torre syndrome is mandatory, so that adequate screening and treatment can be carried out.

15.5.3 Peutz-Jeghers Syndrome

Labial and cutaneous pigmented macules (lentigines) (Fig. 15.81). This autosomal dominant syndrome is related to a mutation of a serine/threonine protein kinase. Patients develop a polyposis of the digestive tract (particularly the jejunum). They have an increased risk of cancers of the digestive tract and also of other organs such as the breast, the pancreas, and the gonads. Lentigines (brown macules), which are predominant on the lips (Fig. 15.81) and oral mucosa, are an easily identifiable cutaneous marker. These lesions appear during childhood and may decrease later on.

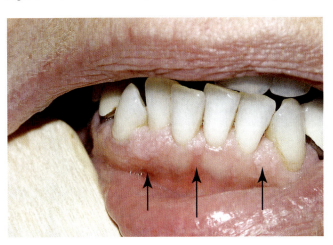

Fig. 15.78

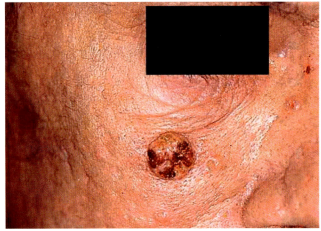

Fig. 15.80

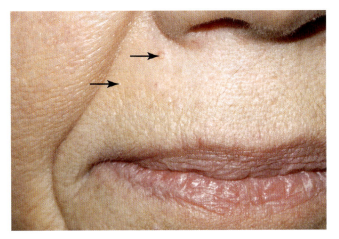

Fig. 15.79

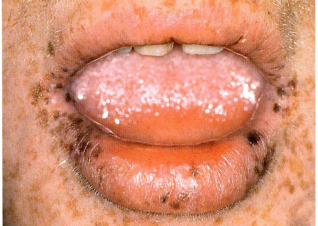

Fig. 15.81

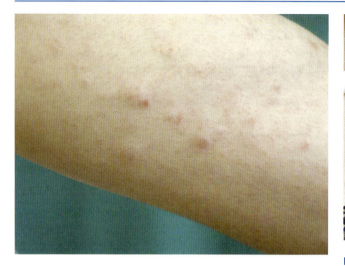

Fig. 15.82

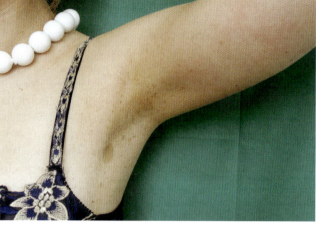

Fig. 15.83

15.5.4 Multiple Leiomyomas: Reed's Syndrome

Multiple flesh-colored or slightly erythematous papules without alteration of the cutaneous surface (Fig. 15.82). Multiple leiomyomas (in a patient with a fumarate-hydratase mutation). Leiomyomas belong to the group of painful skin tumors (cf. page 183, Chap. 30), either spontaneously or on palpation. The cutaneous surface is smooth and non-altered since the tumor is exclusively dermal. Diagnosis is confirmed by skin biopsy. Leiomyomas can be the cutaneous manifestation of a fumarate-hydratase deficiency; in this context, there is an increased risk of kidney cancer and visceral leiomyomas, particularly uterine leiomyomas in women.

15.6   Genetically Determined Diseases

15.6.1 Neurofibromatosis

Café-au-lait spots and mini café-au-lait spots are grouped in the axillary fold (Crowe sign). Von Recklinghausen's neurofibromatosis or NF1 (Fig. 15.83). The presence of one or two café-au-lait spots (CLS) is very common. However, if they are multiple (>6), they can be the cutaneous marker of several genetic diseases, particularly type 1 neurofibromatosis (NF1 or von Recklinghausen's disease). In NF1, café-au-lait spots can be very large (>1.5 cm, sometimes >20 cm) or small (<0.5 cm, often referred to as lentigines) (Figs. 15.83 and 15.84). Their clustered arrangement in the large skin folds is characteristic (Crowe sign, Fig. 15.83). Neurofibromas are almost always present in NF1. They are depressible, flesh-colored or brown papules (cf. Fig. 4.8) of various sizes. Some patients present with deep neurofibromas, which are

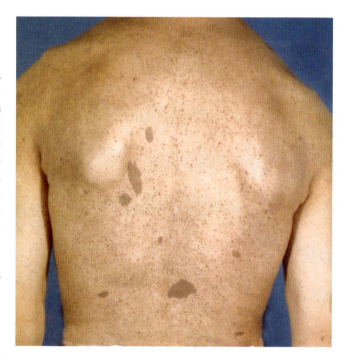

Fig. 15.84

subcutaneous mobile nodules causing skin elevation of normal-looking skin. These patients have a worse prognosis. Also note the deformation of the back, illustrated on Fig. 15.84 as scoliosis is common in this disorder.

15.6.2 Tuberous Sclerosis (Bourneville's Disease)

Multiple flesh-colored or erythematous papules of the face. Angiofibromas (Fig. 15.85). Tuberous sclerosis (or Bourneville's disease) is an autosomal dominant disease

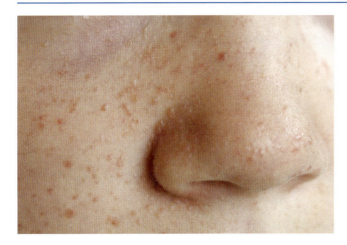

Fig. 15.85

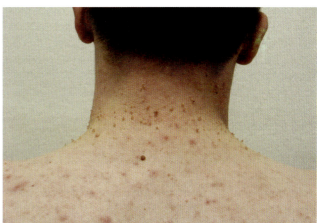

Fig. 15.87

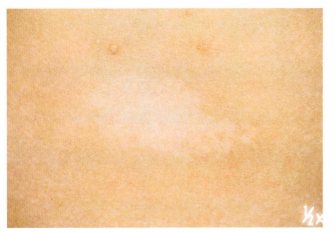

Fig. 15.86

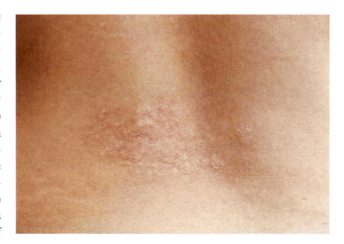

Fig. 15.88

characterized by the onset of numerous benign tumors in the brain (tubers, subependymal tumors), kidneys (angiomyolipomas), and lungs (lymphangioleiomyomatosis). The presence of cardiac rhabdomyomas in the fetus allows prenatal in utero diagnosis using ultrasound; these lesions disappear during the first year. Cutaneous signs are numerous and allow to establish diagnosis: leukodermic macules (Fig. 15.86) with a classical "white leaf" shape (or in the shape of a spade), often present at birth; facial angiofibromas (telangiectatic, millimeter-wide, or larger papules that may become confluent) (Fig. 15.85) occurring during childhood; periungual fibromas known as Koenen tumors (Fig. 15.87, arrow) occurring after adolescence; multiple cervical pendulums (Fig. 15.88); and shagreen patches (Fig. 15.89). Some of these cutaneous signs can also be observed in multiple endocrine neoplasia type 1, which is an important differential diagnosis.

Fig. 15.89

15.6.3 Multiple Endocrine Neoplasias (MEN)

15.6.3.1 MEN Type 1

Multiple flesh-colored papules. Collagenomas, MEN1 (Fig. 15.90, arrows). Multiple endocrine neoplasia type 1 predisposes to adenomas of the pituitary gland (hypophysis), parathyroids, pancreas (VIPoma, glucagonoma, insulinoma, etc.), and adrenal cortex, as well as to Zollinger-Ellison syndrome. From a dermatological point of view, it can mimic a tuberous sclerosis (or Bourneville's disease), since the patients may have multiple facial angiofibromas, leukodermic macules, and collagenomas (Fig. 15.90). These patients also present with lipomas.

15.6.3.2 MEN Type 2B

Multiple mucosal papules and nodules. Neuromas, MEN2B (Fig. 15.91). From a dermatological point of view, it is characterized by multiple mucosal neuromas that are very typical (Fig. 15.91). Patients are often marfanoid (tall size, arachnodactyly, pectus excavatum). They develop medullary thyroid cancer and pheochromocytoma; this is the most aggressive form of MEN.

15.6.4 Pseudoxanthoma Elasticum

Multiple yellow papules that merge to form linear lesions in the cervical area (Fig. 15.92). It is a recessively (or rarely dominantly) transmitted disease, related to the mutation of the gene *ABCC6*. This mutation causes elastorrhexis, which is a fragmentation and thickening of elastic fibers, followed by their abnormal calcification inside the skin, the vessels, and the Bruch's membrane in the eye,

thus causing accelerated atheromatosis and/or hemorrhages of the digestive tract and retina. Cutaneous findings include yellow dermal papules, mostly found on the folds (Fig. 15.92) and mucosa (Fig. 15.93, arrow). Such lesions must be looked for in patients without known cardiovascular

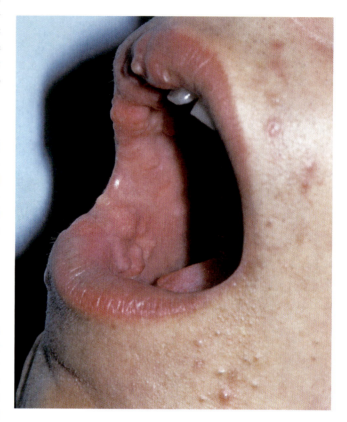

Fig. 15.91

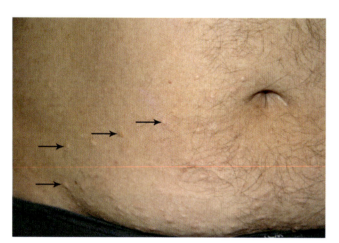

Fig. 15.90

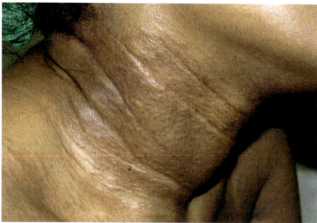

Fig. 15.92

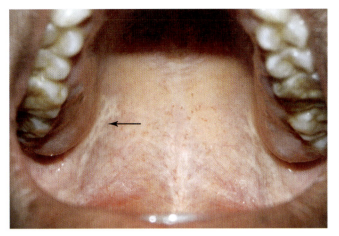

Fig. 15.93

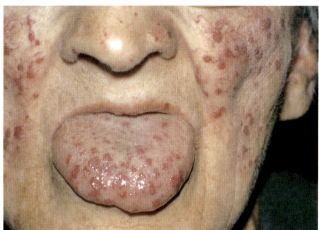

Fig. 15.94

risk factors and who have multiple unexplained vascular events (strokes, myocardial infarction, arteritis of the lower limbs, renovascular hypertension, etc.). A similar clinical phenotype, not related to an *ABCC6* gene mutation, may be associated with a deficiency in vitamin K-dependent coagulation factors.

15.6.5   Rendu-Osler Disease

Multiple cutaneous and mucosal papular telangiectases (Fig. 15.94). This clinical phenotype can be caused by various mutations of the genes involved in the TGF-β transduction pathway. It is characterized by papular telangiectases, particularly on extremities (Fig. 15.95, arrow), lips, and oral mucosa (Fig. 15.94). These patients may have epistaxis and visceral arteriovenous fistulas, particularly in the lungs, which are responsible for the severity of the disease (pulmonary arterial hypertension, right-to-left shunting causing strokes and brain abscesses, etc.). It is an autosomal dominant disease that can be of very late onset (after 50). Telangiectases are often rectangular, as in scleroderma (cf. Fig. 15.27); however, in scleroderma, they remain macular.

15.6.6   Fabry Disease

Multiple millimeter-wide angiomatous papules. Angiokeratomas (Fig. 15.96). Fabry disease is an X-linked metabolic disorder that leads to excessive deposition of globotriaosylceramide in the vascular endothelium of several organs

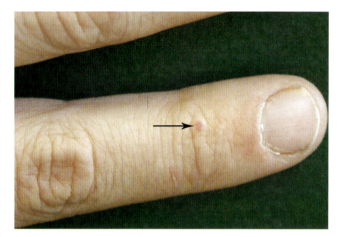

Fig. 15.95

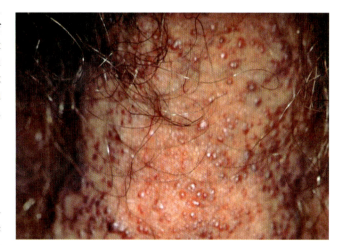

Fig. 15.96

(brain, heart, kidneys, cornea, and skin) and is caused by a deficiency of α-galactosidase A. Dermatological signs are common: lymphedema, hand varicose veins, hypohidrosis, telangiectases, and mainly multiple angiokeratomas characteristically distributed in the swimsuit area (Fig. 15.97). However, the patient in this figure did not have Fabry disease. Diffuse angiokeratoma corporis invariably commands a thorough medical checkup, since several other metabolic overload diseases can manifest in a similar way.

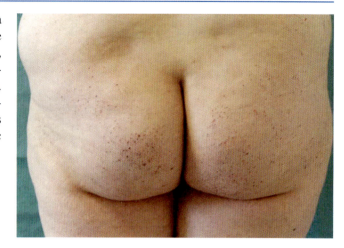

Fig. 15.97

One of the goals of this part is to raise awareness of the spectrum of dermatological differential diagnosis, which includes diseases of various underlying pathomechanisms.

As such, skin may be *affected by external factors* such as inflammatory cells or overload substances. Anomalies may be primarily located inside the skin, as in blaschkolinear inflammatory diseases, although their manifestation and clinical expression are mediated by inflammatory cells. Differential diagnosis should therefore include diseases that result from the following mechanisms:

- *Inflammatory diseases* of multiple causes: genetic, infectious, autoimmune, autoinflammatory, etc.
- *Overload diseases* associated with the deposition of substances that are usually absent from the skin, such as amyloidosis and mucinoses.
- *Diseases due to deprivation of vessels, nerves, or hormones or, on the contrary, due to vessels, nerves, and hormones that are hyper-afferent,* the causes being varied. Thus, obstructive vasculopathies associated with advanced peripheral arterial disease, for instance, result in vascular deprivation, contrarily to arteriovenous malformations, which are responsible for hypervascularization.
- *Diseases caused by physical or chemical trauma.* Diseases that are directly caused by environmental factors are particularly common in dermatology.

The disorder can also be *inherent to the skin*, even if it is secondary to an external factor such as a skin cancer complicating skin aging, an angiosarcoma complicating a lymphedema, or a MALT (mucosa-associated lymphoid tissue)-type lymphoma complicating continuous microbial antigenic stimulation. Such mechanisms underlie the following diseases:

- *Diseases caused by cell proliferation and hypertrophy*, namely, benign tumors and skin cancers.
- *Diseases associated with malformations*, which are numerous, such as clefts and fistulas.
- *Diseases resulting from skin immaturity or, on the contrary, skin degeneration and/or senescence.* In this respect, signs of decline are becoming an increasing reason for consultation, due to population aging and society's demands. Certain aspects of skin aging such as dermatoporosis are a real medical problem.
- *Diseases associated with an inherent functional and/or differentiation disorder*, particularly of the epidermis, such as ichthyoses.
- Diseases for which the lesional mechanism is unknown, mixed, or difficult to classify.

Regardless of the lesional mechanism, the causes of these diseases always come down to the interaction between a mono- or multifactorial genetic predisposition and the environment.

Hence, skin manifestations may appear in diseases that are infectious, tumoral, inflammatory, metabolic, endocrine, toxic, thrombotic, exogenous, and genetic. Therefore, cutaneous signs allow diagnosing as well a mixed connective tissue disease, a systemic vasculitis, or a colon cancer, to name but a very few examples.

It is easy to identify a localized hypopigmented area in a dark-skinned individual. It can however be a difficult task to identify a widespread hypopigmentation in a fair skin individual. The extent of the reduction in pigmentation can be evaluated comparatively with the surrounding healthy skin if it is a localized hypopigmentation, whereas when the whole integument is involved, evaluation is done by comparing with the parents' skin color. In some cases, when the lesions are widespread, it can be difficult to determine whether it is primary a disorder of hyper- or of hypopigmentation. Hence history taking, the effect of tanning, and the inspection of naturally less pigmented areas such as inner arms and buttocks can be helpful. In other areas, lesions may instead be very subtle. Wood's lamp examination may then assist the identification of leukodermas that are due to reduced epidermal melanin content, by enhancing the contrast with normally pigmented skin.

Important clues in establishing diagnosis of a leukoderma are its diffuse or circumscribed nature as well as the age of lesion onset. It is therefore convenient to distinguish between (at least initially) circumscribed leukodermas and diffuse leukodermas: the latter affecting the entire integument, as well as the appendages, and corresponding mainly to the various types of albinism (cf. algorithm, Table 16.1). Other elements essential to the establishment of differential diagnosis are the age of lesion onset, the presence of lesional hyposensitivity (leprosy), family background, and other related signs. Certain particular clinical aspects such as confetti-like or guttate leukodermas (Box 16.1), or blaschkolinear leukodermas (Box 16.2), also help to guide the diagnosis. Lastly, it is essential to specify whether the lesion was straightaway leukodermic or not. When the hypopigmented area was preceded by another lesion, the diagnosis of a postinflammatory hypopigmentation or a regressing tumor is plausible.

Certain infectious or systemic diseases, such as sarcoidosis or leprosy for example, can appear as leukodermic macules that must be purposely biopsied since the histopathological examination will reveal their characteristic appearance. Certain variants of vitiligo are the dermatological manifestation of an uveomeningitis (Vogt-Koyanagi-Harada syndrome)

Table 16.1 Diagnostic approach to leukoderma, according to extension of the lesion (diffuse or localized) and the age of onset

I. Diffuse leukoderma

A. Present at birth or prematurely (childhood)	Albinisms, pigmentary dilution syndrome, phenylketonuria, Menkes syndrome, and related syndromes
	Other rare genetic syndromes (or disorders)
B. Acquired and of later onset	Evolution of an initially circumscribed leukoderma: Vitiligo, chemical leukoderma, malnutrition, hypoparathyroidism, etc.

II. Circumscribed leukoderma

A. Present at birth or prematurely (childhood)	Genetic mosaïcism and nevus depigmentosus
	Tuberous sclerosis (of Bourneville), piebaldism, Waardenburg syndrome
	Other rare genetic syndromes
	Premature onset of a disease that is usually acquired later in life: vitiligo, postinflammatory leukoderma, etc.
B. Of late onset	Vitiligo
	Postinflammatory hypopigmentation: pityriasis lichenoides, subacute lupus erythematosus, etc.
	Infectious hypopigmentations: leprosy, achromic pityriasis versicolor, etc.
	Hypochromic variants of inflammatory diseases which can be characterized histopathologically: sarcoidosis, etc.
	Hypochromic variants of tumors which can be pathologically ascertained: melanoma, atypical nevi, Paget's disease, tumor of the follicular infundibulum, clear cell papulosis, white fibrous papulosis of the neck, white lentiginosis, etc.
	Idiopathic guttate hypomelanosis
	Anemic hamartoma (or nevus anemicus), Bier spots

or of autoimmune polyglandular syndromes. Cutaneous (or tissue) infarction caused by the thrombosing vasculopathy of Köhlmeier-Degos' disease appears as depressed porcelain-white papules that are surrounded by a discreet telangiectatic rim. Their identification allows to correctly diagnose and nosologically classify patients with as to then unexplained cerebral infarction and unresolved pictures of digestive tract surgery. Leukodermic macules (Box 16.3) are often the first sign of tuberous sclerosis.

D. Lipsker, *Clinical Examination and Differential Diagnosis of Skin Lesions*, DOI 10.1007/978-2-8178-0411-8_16, © Springer-Verlag France 2013

Box 16.1 Main Causes of Guttate Leukoderma

Achromic flat warts

Arsenicism (or arsenic poisoning)

Association with various chromosomal abnormalities

Chronic pityriasis lichenoides

Confetti-like lesions in tuberous sclerosis

Darier's disease

Dyschromic amyloidosis

Frictional lichenoid dermatitis

Idiopathic guttate hypomelanosis

Lichen sclerosus (white spot disease)

Multiple endocrine neoplasia, type 1

Pityriasis alba (rarely guttate)

Punctate leukoderma and disseminated hypopigmented keratoses following PUVA therapy

Punctate vitiligo

Systemic sclerosis especially in dark-skinned people

White lentiginosis

Xeroderma pigmentosum

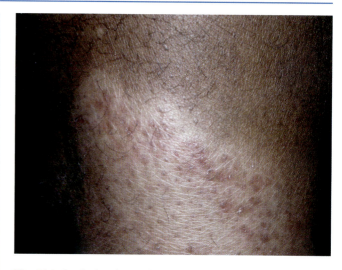

Fig. 16.2 Leukodermic macule. Leprosy. Also note the red millimeter-wide papules. These lesions are hypoesthetic or anesthetic

Box 16.2 Main Causes of Blaschkolinear Leukoderma

Achromic lichen striatus and postinflammatory sequelae of lichen striatus

Association with certain blaschkolinear nevi: epidermal hamartoma, comedo nevus, basaloid follicular hamartoma, etc.

Female carrier of Menkes syndrome

Focal dermal hypoplasia (or Goltz' syndrome)

Incontinentia pigmenti – hypopigmented stage

Ito's hypomelanosis, nevus depigmentosus, and other manifestations of pigmentary mosaicism

Vitiligo (blaschkolinear)

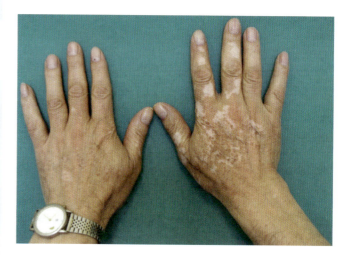

Fig. 16.3 Leukodermic macules on the back of the hands. Vitiligo

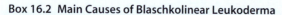
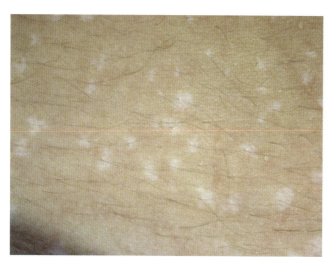

Fig. 16.1 Confetti-like leukoderma

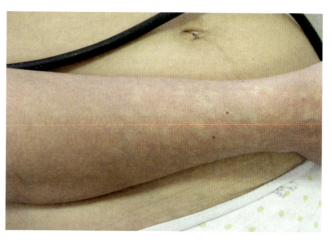

Fig. 16.4 Pale macules on the forearms. Bier spots. These lesions are not pathological. They are increased with venous hyperpressure, for example, when a blood pressure cuff is inflated, between the systolic and diastolic values, as in this example

Box 16.3   Main Causes of Leukodermic Macules

Albinism

Bier spots

Chemically induced hypomelanosis (hydroquinone, phenolic compounds, etc.)

Clear cell papulosis (sometimes macular but mostly papular)

Idiopathic guttate hypomelanosis

Infectious diseases: leprosy, achromic pityriasis versicolor, endemic treponematosis, epidermodysplasia verruciformis

Inflammatory diseases (with characteristic histopathological findings): lichen sclerosus, malignant atrophic papulosis, morphea and pigmentary disorder in systemic sclerosis, sarcoidosis

Ito's hypomelanosis

Livedoid vasculopathy (atrophie blanche)

Mucous membrane leukoplakia

Nevus anemicus

Nevus depigmentosus

Piebaldism and Waardenburg syndrome

Pityriasis alba

Poliosis (hair)

Postinflammatory hypopigmentation

Progressive macular hypomelanosis

Segmental and guttate hypomelanosis with hypermelanocytosis

Tumors: halo nevus and halo melanoma, achromic mycosis fungoides, clinically atypical achromic nevus, tumor of the follicular infundibulum

Vitiligo and associated syndromes (Vogt-Koyanagi-Harada)

White leaf-shaped macules in tuberous sclerosis (Bourneville's disease)

White lentiginosis

White papulosis of the neck

Do Not Miss

In the presence of a white isolated lesion, it is important not to overlook a regressing or achromic melanoma.

Sometimes, mycosis fungoides appears as leukodermic macules, especially in patients with dark skin. Leprosy and sarcoidosis can also appear as hypochromic macules. A guttate leukoderma may reflect arsenicism.

Finally, white spots in a newborn may reveal a tuberous sclerosis or a Waardenburg syndrome.

Common

Pityriasis alba, achromic pityriasis versicolor.

Hyperpigmented Lesions

17

Lesions which are darker than normal skin can be brown, black, or sometimes blue-gray.

The distribution and arrangement of lesions are important semiological elements to be specified, as well as the circumscribed or diffuse nature of the pigmentary disorder. A mucous involvement must also be investigated. Certain topographies are noteworthy.

Circumscribed disorders correspond to macules or pigmented patches that are clearly individualized, whereas diffuse lesions are poorly defined and generally widespread. Pigmentary disorders are often diffuse; they usually first appear and predominate in sun-exposed areas. When a pigmentary disorder is diffuse, it can sometimes be difficult to determine whether the pathological component is the one which is too pigmented or, on the contrary, the one which is lighter. History taking, comparison to naturally less pigmented skin (e.g., inner arms), and comparison to other members of the family can thus be decisive.

Sometimes hyper- and hypopigmented lesions may coexist in what is known as dyschromatosis.

The color of the lesions gives an indication of the type of pigmentary disorder:

- Brown or brown black for epidermal and dermo-epidermal hypermelaninosis.
- Blue or blue-gray, sometimes with a metallic sheen, for dermal melanoses (also known as ceruleoderma) and certain exogenous and endogenous deposits of non-melanin pigments (also known as dyschromia).

In general, the cutaneo-conjunctival yellow coloration of icterus (jaundices), the orange-yellow color which spares the conjunctivae in carotenemias, as well as the ochre, light brown, or reddish brown coloration due to hemosiderin deposits, readily suggests the diagnosis.

The distribution, arrangement, and topography of the lesions provide an important help to diagnosis (Tables 17.1 and 17.2).

Table 17.1 Diagnostic approach to a brown hyperpigmentation (melanoderma) according to the arrangement, distribution and the circumscribed or diffuse nature of a lesion (non-exhaustive list)

Special arrangement	Absence of any notable arrangement
Blaschkolinear hyperpigmentations	*Circumscribed hyperpigmentation, well-defined*
Incontinentia pigmenti	Tumors, hyperplasias, and pigmented hamartomas
McCune-Albright syndrome	Urticaria pigmentosa (mastocytosis)
Linear and whirled nevoid hypermelanosis	Interface dermatitides, often pigmented at advanced stage
Early stage of a verrucous epidermal nevus	Fixed drug eruption
Linear atrophoderma of Moulin	Lichen (planus)
Focal dermal hypoplasia	Ashy dermatosis (of Ramirez)
Partington X-linked cutaneous amyloidosis (in girls)	Others: lupus erythematosus, dermatomyositis, etc.
Segmental neurofibromatosis	Macular amyloidosis
Pigmented sequelae of inflammatory blaschkolinear dermatoses (fixed drug eruption, lichen, psoriasis, etc.)	Acanthosis nigricans
Chimerism	Notalgia paresthetica and frictional pigmentation and other physical causes: radiodermatitis, erythema ab igne (hot water bottle rash), etc.
Other linear pigmentations	Phototoxic reactions: phytophotodermatitis, Berloque dermatitis, Riehl's melanosis, poikiloderma of Civatte, perioral dermatitis
Pigmentary demarcation lines	Idiopathic eruptive pigmentation

(continued)

D. Lipsker, *Clinical Examination and Differential Diagnosis of Skin Lesions*,
DOI 10.1007/978-2-8178-0411-8_17, © Springer-Verlag France 2013

Table 17.1 (continued)

Special arrangement	Absence of any notable arrangement
Pigmentary sequelae of exogenous dermatoses, e.g., phytophotodermatitis	Pigmented variants of certain dermatoses: morphea (atrophoderma of Pasini and Pierini), granuloma annulare, etc.
Pigmented sequelae of linear endogenous dermatoses: lymphangitis, superficial venous thrombosis, zoster, etc.	Pigmented form of mycosis fungoides
Reticulate hyperpigmentation	Pigmented form of common infections: erythrasma, pityriasis versicolor, tinea nigra, etc.
Zinsser-Cole-Engman syndrome	Dermal melanocytosis
Naegeli-Franceschetti-Jadassohn syndrome	Tattoo
Dyschromatoses (universalis hereditaria, acropigmentation of Dohi)	Postinflammatory pigmentation
Dermatopathia pigmentosa reticularis	*Diffuse hyperpigmentation, poorly defined, photo-exposed, or generalized*
Dowling-Degos disease	Hypermelaninosis
Reticulate acropigmentation of Kitamura	Metabolic and overload
Confluent and reticulated papillomatosis of Gougerot and Carteaud	Hemochromatosis (hemosiderosis and hypermelaninosis)
Partington-type X-linked cutaneous amyloidosis (in boys)	Porphyrias
Mendes da Costa syndrome	Cirrhoses
Weary-Kindler syndrome	Renal impairment
Metameric reticulate hyperpigmentation	Generalized macular amyloidosis
Revesz's syndrome	Other rare diseases: Wilson's disease, Gaucher's disease, Niemann-Pick's disease, lipoproteinosis
Erythema ab igne	Endocrine
Pigmented sequelae of inflammatory reticulate dermatoses (i.e., inflammatory livedo from polyarteritis nodosa, prurigo pigmentosa)	Addison's disease, Cushing syndrome, and other endocrinopathies (hyperthyroidism, acromegaly, Nelson's syndrome, etc.)
Flagellated hyperpigmentations	Ectopic secretion or therapeutic administration of ACTH or MSH
Dermatomyositis	Pheochromocytoma and carcinoid
Toxic: bleomycin, mushroom, shiitake, etc.	Pregnancy, chloasma
	Deficiencies and malabsorption
	Pellagra and pellagroid syndromes
	Vitamin deficiencies: B12, folates, vitamins C and A
	Whipple's disease and celiac disease
	Kwashiorkor
	Physical
	Drug-induced or toxic (e.g., arsenic): antimalarials, minocycline, phenothiazines, etc.
	Chronic infections
	Endocarditis
	Parasitoses
	HIV infection
	Tuberculosis, malaria, etc.
	Tumoral and during blood disorders
	Metastatic melanoma
	Sézary's syndrome and other blood disorders
	POEMS syndrome, scleredema, etc.
	Diencephalic tumors
	Neurological, particularly diseases affecting the diencephalon
	Systemic diseases and plasma cell proliferations: Still's disease, rheumatoid arthritis, lupus erythematosus, sclerodermas, POEMS syndrome, Gleich's syndrome, H syndrome, etc.
	Genetical
	Congenital diffuse melanocytosis
	Zanardo's syndrome
	Hemosiderosis
	Dyschromia

ACTH adrenocorticotropic hormone, *MSH* melanocyte-stimulating hormone, *POEMS* polyneuropathy, organomegaly, endocrinopathy, monoclonal component, skin lesion

Table 17.2 Causes of hyperpigmentations according to their topography

Facial pigmentations	Chloasma
	Drug eruption (hydantoin, amiodarone, etc.)
	Exogenous ochronosis (hydroquinone)
	Gaucher's disease
	HIV infection
	Hyperthyroidism
	Initial stage of diffuse addisonian hyperpigmentations
	Pellagra
	Perioral dermatitis
	Poikiloderma of Civatte
	Porphyria
	Riehl's melanosis
Pigmentation of folds	Acanthosis nigricans
	Chromhidrosis
	Dowling-Degos disease
	Gougerot-Carteaud syndrome
	Initial stage of dermatopathia pigmentosa reticularis
	Lichen planus
	Weary-Kindler syndrome
Pigmentation of the oral cavity	*External causes:* tattooing by dental amalgams, metal deposits (lead, bismuth, arsenic, etc.)
	Drug eruption (fixed drug eruption and deposits): antimalarials, minocycline, etc.
	Oral hyperpigmentation in general diseases: Addison's disease, hemochromatosis, HIV infection, chronic lung diseases and bronchial carcinomas, etc.
	Genetical: lentigines in Peutz-Jeghers syndrome, Laugier-Hunziker's syndrome
	Acquired tumors: melanoma, nevus
	Inflammations: melanoacanthoma, postinflammatory hyperpigmentation (lichen, etc.)

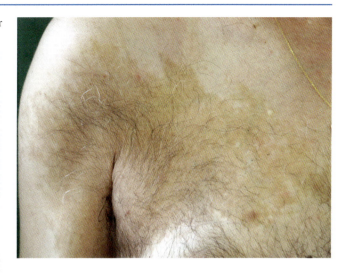

Fig. 17.1 Irregular and hairy café-au-lait macule. Becker's nevus. Becker's nevus usually becomes apparent at puberty. Sometimes, it can be associated with a hypotrophy of the homolateral limb and a mammary hyoplasia in the context of a Becker's nevus syndrome

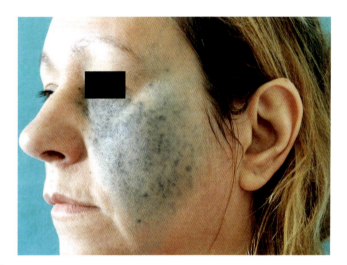

Fig. 17.2 Bluish-grey macule, called ceruleodermic, of V-2 territory. Nevus of Ota. This type of nevus can become complicated with glaucoma and rarely with a melanoma. It was the case with this patient who had developed a melanoma of fatal evolution on the nevus of Ota. Note also the inhomogeneous character of the pigmentation with several darker areas, sometimes papular and palpable

Thus, most genetically determined hyperpigmentations appear in childhood, are generally circumscribed or figurate and well demarcated, and can be integrated into a polymalformative syndrome. Acquired hyperpigmentations occur more readily in adults, are often poorly defined and widespread, and result from multiple causes particularly metabolic, endocrine, and drug toxicity. Adrenal insufficiency, hemochromatosis, POEMS syndrome, and Whipple's disease are examples of systemic diseases for which hyperpigmentation may be one of their cutaneous manifestations.

Finally, all palpable cutaneous lesions can be pigmented and they will thus be addressed in the corresponding chapter.

Table 17.3 Main causes of pigmented macules	Brown or black macule	Necrosis (differential diagnosis)
		Alkaptonuria (ochronosis and hydroquinone-acquired ochronosis)
		Chloasma (melasma)
		Confluent and reticulate papillomatosis of Gougerot and Carteaud
		Dermal melanocytoses (Mongolian spot, nevus of Ota and of Ito) and plaque-type blue nevus
		Diabetic dermopathy
		Dowling-Degos disease and acropigmentation of Kitamura
		Drug eruption
		Early stage of generalized hyperpigmentations
		Fixed drug eruption
		Gaucher's disease and Niemann-Pick's disease
		Granulomatous diseases: granuloma annulare and necrobiosis lipoidica
		Histologically characterized inflammatory diseases: lichen planus, lupus erythematosus, morphea, and scleroderma (atrophoderma of Pasini and Pierini)
		Hyperthyroidism
		Idiopathic eruptive pigmentation
		Incontinentia pigmenti (late stage)
		Infectious diseases: dermatophytosis nigricans, erythrasma, and pityriasis versicolor
		Metabolic and overload diseases: macular amyloidosis and lipoproteinosis
		Notalgia paresthetica
		Phytophotodermatitis (Berloque dermatitis)
		Pigmentary demarcation line
		Pigmentation of venous insufficiency
		Pigmented mycosis fungoides
		Postinflammatory melanoderma
		Tumors and hamartomas: melanoma, nevus, nevus spilus, lentigo, seborrheic keratosis, linear epidermal hamartoma, Becker's nevus, café au lait spot, etc.
		Urticaria pigmentosa
	Blue or gray macule	Argyria
		Ashy dermatosis of Ramirez
		Cutaneous osteoma
		Endemic treponematosis
		Hemochromatosis
		Mongolian spot
		Metastatic melanoma with melanuria
		Neurocutaneous melanosis
		Nevus of Ota and Ito and other acquired dermal melanocytoses (of the extremities and the back, during NF1, etc.)
		Periorbital heliotrope erythema of dermatomyositis
		Postinflammatory melanoderma, tattoo (lead, graphite, tar, carbon, etc.), and injection of ferrous salts
		Venous lake (particularly on the lips and the ears)

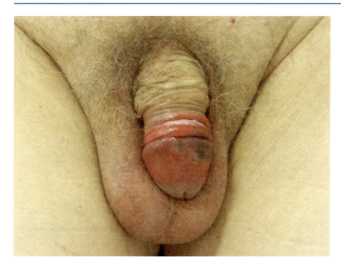

Fig. 17.3 Blueish-gray macule in an erosive balanoposthitis. Zoon's balanoposthitis. The coloration is due to iron deposit in this chronic and benign inflammatory disorder

Do Not Miss

Unique pigmented lesion: consider melanoma and other pigmented malignant tumors.

Diffuse and/or generalized hyperpigmentations: consider a general disorder (endocrine, metabolic, and systemic diseases).

Common

Poikiloderma of Civatte and dermatoheliosis.

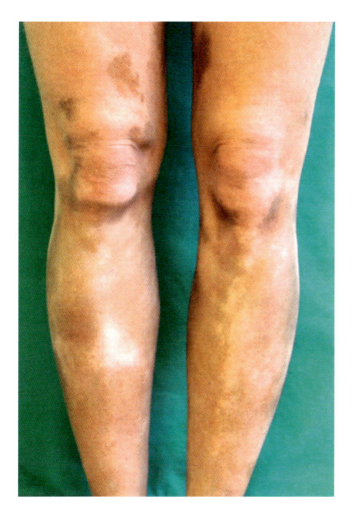

Fig. 17.4 Pigmented patches. Pigmented purpuric dermatosis (Schamberg's disease)

The intensity of an erythema depends on the room temperature where the patient is being examined and on the patient's position, whether lying or standing, which explains its variability. For example, in certain angiosarcomas of the face, erythema becomes apparent only when the patient tilts her head downwards for 1 min (known as tilt test). Erythema can be permanent or paroxysmal. It can display a notable configuration, annular or grid-like (livedo). Numerous tones of red (ranging from pink to violet) exist and are of great semiological value to the experimented physician in the orientation of diagnosis. The association of erythema, pain, edema, and increased temperature is characteristic of inflammation in the broad sense. Erythemas of the folds (also known as intertrigo), the extremities, the face, the scrotum, or the buttocks in children often have specific causes and are covered in Chap. 19. Causes of exanthemas are covered in Chap. 20 and causes of erythroderma are summarized in Chap. 21.

Erythema can be the superficial cutaneous expression of an inflammation of infectious or tumoral origin, located within an underlying anatomical structure. Such a cause should not be overlooked. Erythema is also one of the first and sometimes the only symptom of several cutaneous infections such as erysipelas, zoster, or erythema migrans caused by infection with *Borrelia burgdorferi*, for example. Lastly, several systemic diseases called "auto-inflammatory disorders," or generally speaking which involve a dysfunction of innate immunity, manifest as erythematous lesions of sudden onset which are often accompanied by fever and subside within a few hours or days.

Box 18.1 Main Causes of Red Macules

External causes: friction, burn, sunburn, etc.

Fixed drug eruption

Follicular mucinosis (usually squamous)

Granulomatous diseases: granuloma annulare, interstitial granulomatous dermatitis

Infectious diseases: erythema migrans, acrodermatitis chronica atrophicans, erysipela, erysipelothrix infection, tinea incognito, African trypanosomiasis, leprosy, pityriasis versicolor

Inflammation by contiguity (contiguous inflammation of the skin): erythema is situated above an underlying inflammatory disease which is primarily extracutaneous (affecting, e.g., the fascia, muscles, joints, bones, and sinus), e.g., erythema located next to a joint surface in arthritis (gout+++), above underlying fasciitis or ethmoiditis, above a solitary plasmacytoma of bone or a metal implant

Inflammatory diseases: morphea, REM (reticular erythematous mucinosis) syndrome

Inflammatory flare-ups in systemic diseases: Behçet's disease, familial Mediterranean fever (periodic disease), hyper-IgD syndrome (mevalonate kinase deficiency), TRAPS syndrome, hypereosinophilic syndrome, etc.

Initial stage of an infectious cutaneous disease: zoster, herpes, etc.

Initial stage of certain noninfectious dermatoses: pemphigoid, eczema, etc.

Miscellaneous: acrokeratosis paraneoplastica (particularly in its vascular variant), angiomas, reactive angioendotheliomatosis, angiosarcoma, erythrokeratodermia variabilis, initial stage of livedo

Mycosis fungoides (usually squamous)

Necrolytic acral erythema

Recurring scarlatiniform erythema of Féréol-Besnier

D. Lipsker, *Clinical Examination and Differential Diagnosis of Skin Lesions*,
DOI 10.1007/978-2-8178-0411-8_18, © Springer-Verlag France 2013

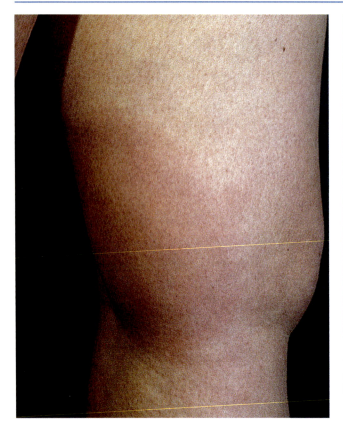

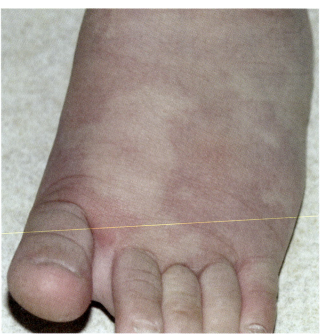

Fig. 18.3   Red angiomatous macule of the back of the foot. Capillary malformation in the context of a Klippel-Trénaunay syndrome; limb hypertrophy was also present

Fig. 18.1   Oval red macule. Erythema migrans caused by infection with *Borrelia burgdorferi*. The progressive extension is characteristic

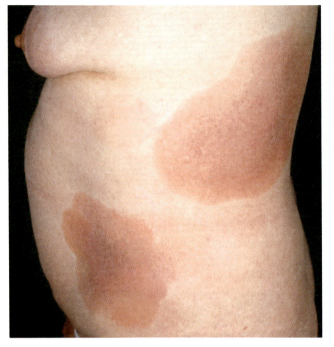

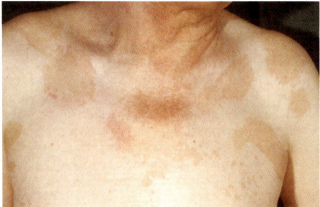

Fig. 18.4   Orange-red macules of the trunk. Pityriasis versicolor. Also note the cervical and presternal telangiectasias related to skin aging

Fig. 18.2   Orange-red macules. Mycosis fungoides. Note the very sharp demarcation of the lesions. Any lasting fixed erythematous macule, with or without anomaly of the cutaneous surface (scaling, atrophy), should suggest this diagnosis

Do Not Miss

Keep in mind contiguous inflammation of the skin (related to inflammation or infection of an underlying anatomical structure, e.g., ethmoiditis, cavernous sinus thrombosis, arthritis), infectious diseases (erysipela, fasciitis, borreliosis, etc.), systemic inflammatory flare-ups (periodic disease and other autoinflammatory diseases, Behçet's disease, hypereosinophilic syndrome), initial stages of certain diseases (herpes, zoster, pemphigoid, etc.), mycosis fungoides, follicular mucinosis, vascular forms of Bazex acrokeratosis, and angiosarcomas.

Common

External causes (burns, friction, etc.). Infections (erysipela, erythema migrans, herpes, pityriasis versicolor). Drug eruption.

19.1 Erythematous Lesions of the Face

Red lesions of the face are common. A midfacial telangiectatic erythema which spares the mobile areas such as the eyelids and lips is typical of rosacea. A scaly erythema in areas rich in sebum, around the eyebrows, glabella, and nasolabial folds, is characteristic of seborrheic dermatitis. These two disorders, along with acne, are the most common causes of facial dermatitis, with a prevalence of 2–4 %. However, several other diseases can cause facial erythema. Flushing accompanied by facial erythema must be distinguished from permanent erythema. Certain paroxysmal erythemas have a special topography which gives an etiological orientation, e.g., hemifacial erythema in Harlequin syndrome points to an injury of the second sympathetic ganglion. Other erythemas appear in particular circumstances such as during meals and can be accompanied by hyperhidrosis as in Frey's syndrome, following injury of the auriculotemporal nerve and anomalous regeneration of the sympathetic fibers that supply the sweat glands instead of the parotid. The timing can also be suggestive, as in postprandial erythema occurring in a dumping syndrome, which is a classic complication of esophagogastric surgery. Onset related to certain characteristic circumstances can give a clue to diagnosis, such as cold temperature (cryoproteins) or hot temperature (red ear syndrome, a variant of erythermalgia) or certain drugs. Permanent, nonparoxysmal lesions must be classified according to their onset, which can be either sudden or progressive. It is essential to determine the presence of associated cutaneous lesions through physical examination: pustules, papules, plaques, and extracutaneous signs, particularly fever or chills, and joint pain. Sometimes, only history taking can reveal the existence of associated lesions, since these may not be present during examination. It is important to specify whether the lesions are photo-induced and/or photo-exposed (cf. Chap. 10). Chondritis may be the consequence of an inflammation of the cartilage, thus causing erythema in cartilaginous areas such as nose wings or pinna while sparing the lobule. Causes of erythematous papules and plaques of the face will be summarized here for teaching purposes.

Table 19.1 Main causes of facial erythema

Nature of lesions	Main causes
Paroxysmal erythema	Blood disorders (i.e., polycythemia)
	Carcinoid syndrome
	Cryoglobulinemia
	Dengue and other arbovirus infections (sunburn appearance)
	Drugs: nicotinic acid, amyl nitrite, disulfiram + alcohol, tacrolimus (topical route), etc.
	Dumping syndrome
	Endocrine tumors of the pancreas
	Erythema pudoris
	Familial dysautonomia, also known as Riley-Day syndrome
	Frey's syndrome
	Hemifacial flushing (Harlequin syndrome) due to injury of the second sympathetic ganglion
	Homocystinuria
	Hyperthyroidism
	Hypoglycemia
	Mastocytosis
	Medullary thyroid cancer
	Menopause
	Pheochromocytoma
	Red ear syndrome
	Rosacea
	Staphylococcal toxic shock syndrome (sunburn appearance)
	Toxic: trichlorethylene, calcium cyanamide, etc.
	Urticaria-like follicular mucinosis

(continued)

D. Lipsker, *Clinical Examination and Differential Diagnosis of Skin Lesions*,
DOI 10.1007/978-2-8178-0411-8_19, © Springer-Verlag France 2013

Table 19.1 (continued)

Nature of lesions	Main causes
Permanent erythema	Acrokeratosis paraneoplastica
	Acute eczema of the face
	Angiosarcoma
	Chondritis (any cause)
	Circumoral dermatitis
	Cushing syndrome
	Dermatomyositis
	Dermatophytosis
	Hemifacial "blue cellulitis" caused by infection with *Haemophilus influenzae* (rarely *pneumococcus*), in infants and children
	Seborrheic dermatitis
	Solar erythema (sunburn)
	Actinic prurigo (mostly found in the mestizo population)
	Chronic carcinoid syndrome
	Contiguous inflammation of the skin: ethmoiditis, sinusitis
	Eosinophilic pustular folliculitis
	Erythema infectiosum (fifth disease, megalerythema epidemicum, and other exanthemas)
	Facial leiomyoma
	Haber's syndrome
	Homocystinuria
	Infant:
	Neonatal lupus erythematosus
	Bloom syndrome
	Rothmund-Thomson syndrome
	Infectious diseases: facial malignant staphylococcal infection, erysipela, zoster or herpes, etc.
	Leprosy
	Lupus erythematosus
	Lupus vulgaris
	Lysinuric protein intolerance, lysinuria (neonatal pseudolupus)
	Multicentric reticulohistiocytosis (dermatomyositis-like)
	Mycosis fungoides
	Pellagra, vitamins B2 and B6 deficiency
	Polycythemia
	Polymorphous light eruption
	Rosacea
	Sarcoidosis ("lupus pernio," "angiolupoid")
	Sebopsoriasis
	Seborrheic pemphigus
	Superior vena cava syndrome
	Ulerythema ophryogenes
	Urticaria-like follicular mucinosis
Erythematous papule(s) and/or plaque(s)	Acne
	Angiosarcoma
	Annular erythema in Sjögren syndrome
	Dermatomyositis
	Dermatophytosis
	Eczema/dermatitis (contact, photoallergic, aeroallergic, atopic, etc.)
	Erythema multiforme
	Seborrheic dermatitis
	Angiolymphoid hyperplasia with eosinophilia
	Chilblain lupus erythematosus of Hutchinson
	Erysipela and facial malignant staphylococcal infection
	Graft-versus-host reaction
	Granuloma faciale (Lever type)
	Idiopathic facial aseptic granuloma
	Jessner-Kanof disease (cutaneous lupus erythematosus)
	Kimura disease
	Leishmaniasis
	Leprosy
	Lupus erythematosus
	Lupus vulgaris Lymphoma
	Melkersson-Rosenthal syndrome
	Pemphigus erythematosus
	Polymorphous light eruption
	Pseudolymphoma caused by infection with *Borrelia*
	Rosacea
	Sarcoidosis (lupus pernio, angiolupoid, pseudolymphoma of Spiegler and Fendt)
	Urticaria-like follicular mucinosis
	Zoster or prevesicular herpes zoster

Paroxysmal Erythema

Paroxysmal erythema may reveal an endocrine tumor that is either benign (pheochromocytoma, carcinoid) or malignant (medullary thyroid cancer). It can be a sign of hypoglycemia. It should not be mistaken for the facial "sunburn" appearance of sudden onset that can be observed in staphylococcal toxic shock syndrome, dengue, and other arbovirus infections.

Common

Flushing in rosacea.

Permanent Erythema

When it is of sudden onset, an infectious cause must be considered first: erysipela, facial malignant staphylococcal infection, infection with *Haemophilus influenzae* in infants, and initial stage of zoster, but also staphylococcal toxic shock syndrome, dengue, and other arbovirus infections. Facial erythema as contiguous inflammation of the skin, in the context of a sinusitis or an ethmoiditis, can be of sudden or progressive onset. Facial erythema is also a common sign in lupus erythematosus or dermatomyositis. An infiltrated and/or violaceous erythema of the face is often the first manifestation of an angiosarcoma. A keratotic erythema which first affects the helix and nose should suggest acrokeratosis paraneoplastica. A superior vena cava syndrome is usually more edematous than erythematous.

Common

Rosacea and seborrheic dermatitis

Palpable Lesions

Erysipela and other infections can manifest as plaques, particularly on the face. Angiosarcoma must always be suspected as well as other cancers such as achromic melanoma or cutaneous carcinomas, especially when lesions are ulcerated and/or crusted.

Lupus erythematosus, pseudolymphoma, and sarcoidosis are often located on the face.

Common

Acne, rosacea

19.2 Palmar and/or Palmoplantar Erythema

Permanent red lesions must be distinguished from paroxysmal phenomena that are triggered by cold temperatures, such as Raynaud's phenomenon, or by hot temperatures, such as erythermalgia. For teaching purposes and to avoid significant overlapping, the causes of plane and palpable red lesions are summarized in the same table. Some diseases which are initially erythematous can evolve towards cyanosis (blue appearance) followed by necrosis and ulceration. Clinicians should not forget to carefully examine the nails and to look for flame-shaped hemorrhages and/or periungual mega-capillaries. They should also be able to recognize scleroderma's palmar telangiectasias that may initially be discreet and are often rectangular.

Table 19.2 Main causes of acral erythema

Nature of the lesion	Main causes
Erythema	Acral erythema (caused by chemotherapy)
	Acrodynia and toxic erythema
	Acrokeratosis paraneoplastica
	Aicardi-Goutieres syndrome
	Chilblain
	Cold agglutinin-induced disease
	Cytomegalovirus infection
	Erysipeloid and other inoculation diseases
	Erythema nodosum of the palms and soles
	Erythermalgia
	Frostbite
	Hepatitis C
	Inherited
	Kawasaki disease
	Liver disease
	Lupus erythematosus
	Pregnancy
	Recurrent perineal erythema
	Scarlatiniform scaled erythema Féréol-Besnier
	Delayed pressure urticaria
	Gloves and socks syndrome (parvovirus B19, EBV, and other viruses)
	HIV
	Neurovascular instability syndrome
	Peeling skin syndrome (acral form)
	Rombo syndrome
	Scarlet fever
	Staphylococcal toxic shock syndrome
	Vasculitis

(continued)

Table 19.2 (continued)

Nature of the lesion	Main causes
Raynaud's phenomenon	Aicardi-Goutieres syndrome
	Angiocentric lymphoma
	Anorexia nervosa
	Autoimmune diseases: scleroderma, mixed connective tissue disease, lupus erythematosus, dermatomyositis (particularly antisynthetase syndrome), rheumatoid arthritis, etc.
	Buerger's disease
	Cannabis-induced arteritis
	Cold agglutinin-induced disease
	Cryoglobulinemia, cryofibrinogenemia
	Drugs and toxic products: polyvinyl chloride, silicone implant, bleomycin, interferon, cyclosporin, COX-2 inhibitors + APL, cocaine, snake bite, etc.
	Ergotism
	Hypereosinophilic syndrome
	Mechanical causes: thoracic outlet syndrome, carpal tunnel syndrome
	Neurovascular instability syndrome
	Raynaud's disease
	Vascular form of acrokeratosis paraneoplastica
	Vascular form of multiple sclerosis
	Virus infections: HIV, parvovirus B19, etc.
Erythermalgia	Connective tissue diseases
	Drugs
	Gout
	Idiopathic
	Multiple sclerosis
	Myeloproliferative syndrome
	Neuropathies, including of small fibers
	Thrombotic thrombocytopenic purpura
	Vasculitis

CMV cytomegalovirus, *EBV* Epstein-Barr virus, *HIV* human immunodeficiency virus

Erythema

Acute erythema should suggest an infectious disease such as staphylococcal toxic shock syndrome or Kawasaki disease but also erysipeloid or infection with *Streptococcus iniae*, as well as other inoculation diseases.

Toxic causes should not be forgotten (mercury, chemotherapy), as well as metabolic and paraneoplastic causes (acrokeratosis paraneoplastica, necrolytic acral erythema of glucagonoma) and chronic viral infections (HIV, HCV [hepatitis C virus]).

In connective tissue diseases, hands are often affected, particularly in lupus erythematosus and dermatomyositis.

Phlebitis and lymphedema are more edematous than erythematous.

Common

Physiological, pregnancy, cirrhosis

Raynaud's Phenomenon

In case of unilateral Raynaud's phenomenon, a compression (thoracic outlet syndrome, carpal tunnel syndrome) should be suspected. If bilateral, toxic causes, connective tissue diseases, and cryopathies must be searched for, and the possibilities of acrokeratosis paraneoplastica and polymyositis, which are often hallmarked by a severe Raynaud's phenomenon, not forgotten.

Common

Raynaud's disease

19.3   Diaper Rash

Examination should specify:

- Topography: friction area, perianal, and predominance in folds
- Associated lesions: papules, erosive and/or crusted papules that should suggest Langerhans cell histiocytosis, pustules that are common in candidiasis, collarette scaling suggesting candidiasis or necrolytic migratory erythema, and bullae (congenital syphilis)
- General signs

Box 19.1 Main Causes of Diaper Rash in Infants

Allergic contact dermatitis (diapers, topical products)
Atopic dermatitis
Candidiasis
Dermatitis herpetiformis
Dermatophytosis
Ecthyma gangrenosum
Gianotti-Crosti syndrome (infantile papular acrodermatitis)
Gluteal granuloma
Irritant dermatitis (contact, "systemic": tooth eruption)
Jacquet's erosive diaper dermatitis (or syphiloid post-erosive pyodermitis of Sevestre and Jacquet)
Kawasaki disease (involvement of the buttocks is common, but there are always associated signs)
Langerhans cell histiocytosis
Necrolytic migratory erythema (enteropathic acrodermatitis)
Psoriasis (napkin psoriasis)
Seborrheic dermatitis (Leiner-Moussous)
Staphylococcal scalded skin syndrome (affection can be predominant on the buttocks, with typical superficial skin detachment)
Streptococcal anitis

19.4   Scrotal Erythema/Edema

Box 19.2 Main Causes of Scrotal Erythema/Edema

Anasarca

Acute urinary retention

Crohn's disease

Erysipela

Fournier's gangrene

Glucagonoma syndrome

Idiopathic scrotal edema in children

Inflammatory flare-up of lymphedema

Neoplastic lymphangitis

Zinc deficiency, vitamin B2 (riboflavin) deficiency, etc.

19.5   Intertrigo

Box 19.3 Main Causes of Intertrigo

Amicrobial pustulosis of the folds

Bacterial intertrigo

Candidiasis

Contact dermatitis and atopic dermatitis

Crohn's disease[a]

Darier's disease

Dermatophytosis

Endogenous eczema and drug eruptions ("SDRIFE")

Erythrasma

Fox-Fordyce's disease[a]

Granular parakeratosis

Hailey-Hailey disease

Hereditary mucoepithelial dysplasia

Hidradenitis suppurativa (acne inverse or Verneuil's disease in the French terminology)

Hyperimmunoglobulin E syndrome (Job syndrome)

Inflammatory adenopathies[a]

Inflammatory apocrine adenocarcinoma[a]

Irritation, maceration

Langerhans cell hystiocytosis[a]

Lichen (planus)

Mycosis fungoides (granulomatous slack skin)

Necrolytic migratory erythema in glucagonoma syndrome, enteropathic acrodermatitis, and related disorders

Olmsted syndrome

Paget's disease[a]

Pemphigus vegetans

Primary HIV infection

Pseudoxanthoma elasticum[a]

Psoriasis

Subcorneal pustulosis of Sneddon-Wilkinson and IgA pemphigus

X-linked ectodermal dysplasia with immunodeficiency (hypomorphic mutations in IKBKG)

[a]Lesions are preferentially located in folds and are not necessarily erythematous; other primary lesions may be associated to erythema: papules, plaques, vesicles, and pustules

Do Not Miss

Some certain serious diseases can manifest as intertrigo: Langerhans cell histiocytosis, glucagonoma syndrome, and pemphigus. Primary HIV infection can manifest as an intertrigo. Simultaneous affection of several folds is characteristic of a particular form of drug eruption.

Common

Maceration (particularly submammary and abdominal folds), atopic dermatitis, bacterial intertrigo, dermatophytosis, candidiasis, and psoriasis

20.1 Maculopapular Exanthema

There are many types of maculopapular exanthema which require an excellent knowledge of nosology and a great experience in order to make a diagnosis. It is essential to perform an in-depth analysis of the associated signs (forewarning signs, influenza-like symptoms, enlarged lymph nodes, enanthema), of the comorbidity, and a drug history. As such, exanthema from measles is maculopapular and confluent while leaving intervals of unaffected skin. It starts from behind the ears and shows a downward progression in a child or adult affected by an oculonasal catarrh, with alteration of the general condition. Its primary lesion is a folliculitis or a perifollicular erythema. The presence of a characteristic associated enanthema (Koplik's sign) enables diagnosis. The exanthema from Still's disease is transient and consists of macules and pink plaques that are barely palpable and particularly located on the trunk. It occurs in the late afternoon during febrile peaks. The associated signs, joint pains, cervical adenopathy, pharyngitis, inflammatory syndrome, leukocytosis, and hepatitis, hold a high diagnostic value.

While drug-induced exanthemas can be pruritic, most infectious exanthemas are not. A confluent erythema, localized or generalized, with edema of the extremities and a marked enanthema, is common in superantigen diseases such as scarlet fever, staphylococcal toxic shock syndrome, or Kawasaki disease. The onset of Lyell's syndrome must be feared in the presence of a macular exanthema evolving towards skin detachment that requires to be thoroughly searched by traction of the skin.

For teaching purposes and in spite of the great value of the nature of the primary lesion, papular and vesicular exanthema are also addressed in this chapter, because they represent a true differential diagnosis on account of their eruptive nature.

Table 20.1 Main causes of maculopapular exanthema[a]

Diagnostic categories	Main causes
Viral diseases	Adenovirus
	CMV
	EBV
	Enterovirus (echovirus, Coxsackie virus, etc.)
	Hepatitis B
	HHV-6
	Measles
	Parvovirus B19
	Primary HIV infection (often roseola with mucous signs)
	Respiratory syncytial virus
	Rubella
Drug eruptions[b]	Antibiotics, anticonvulsants, etc.
Toxin-mediated diseases	Leptospirosis
	Pharyngitis related to *Arcanobacterium haemolyticum*
	Recurring scarlatiniform scaled erythema Féréol-Besnier
	Streptococcal and staphylococcal scarlatina
	Toxic shock syndrome

(continued)

D. Lipsker, *Clinical Examination and Differential Diagnosis of Skin Lesions*,
DOI 10.1007/978-2-8178-0411-8_20, © Springer-Verlag France 2013

Table 20.1 (continued)

Diagnostic categories	Main causes
Others	Acute lupus erythematosus
	Angioimmunoblastic lymphadenopathy
	Graft versus host reaction
	Infections:
	Anaplasmosis (ehrlichiosis)
	Brucellosis
	Chronic meningococcemia and meningitis due to *meningococci*
	Gram-negative bacilli (*Escherichia coli, Klebsiella pneumoniae*, etc.) and other bacteria
	Listeria monocytogenes
	Rat-bite fever
	Recurring fever
	Rickettsiosis (look for the inoculation eschar)
	Salmonellosis
	Secondary syphilis
	Toxoplasmosis
	Typhus
	Kawasaki disease
	Syndrome of lymphocyte recovery

CMV cytomegalovirus, *EBV* Epstein-Barr virus, *HHV-6* human herpesvirus 6, *HIV* human immunodeficiency virus

[a]Must be distinguished from urticaria; some classify the rashes of adult-onset Still's disease and of Schnitzler's syndrome as maculopapular exanthema: however, it is an urticarial rash corresponding mostly to a neutrophilic urticarial dermatosis

[b]Possible evolution towards DRESS (drug reaction with eosinophilia and systemic signs) or erythroderma; early stage of acute exanthematous pustulosis

Do Not Miss

In some cases, the diagnosis of a maculopapular exanthema is real emergency because it may indicate a serious underlying infection (meningitis, septicemia [due to *meningococcus, Salmonella, Rickettsia*, etc.], primary HIV infection, early-stage staphylococcal epidermolysis) and *a toxinic and/or superantigen-mediated* disease (Kawasaki disease, streptococcal toxic shock syndrome, leptospirosis), and it may be the first sign of a serious drug eruption (Lyell's syndrome, acute generalized exanthematous pustulosis, DRESS). Angioimmunoblastic lymphadenopathy and lymphomatoid granulomatosis (Liebow's disease) can also be revealed by a maculopapular exanthema.

Common

Viral exanthema (children, young adults) and drug eruption (adults).

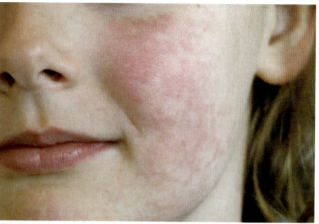
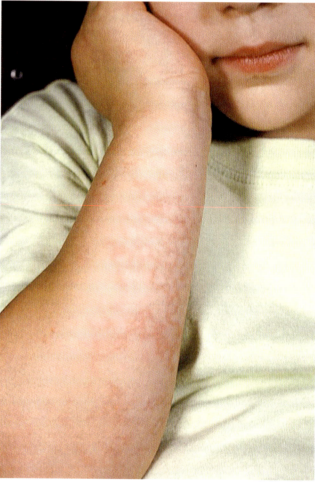

Fig. 20.1 Exanthema with a slapped cheek appearance and characteristic reticulated erythema on the limbs. Primary infection with parvovirus B19 (erythema infectiosum, fifth disease)

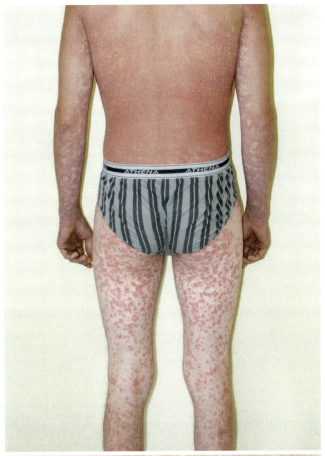

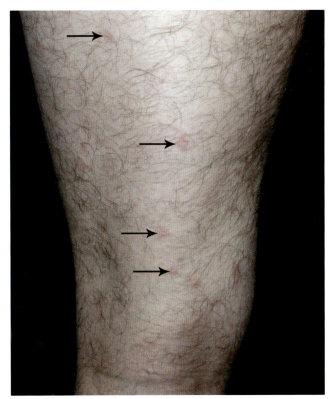

Fig. 20.3 Roseola (*arrows*). Primary HIV infection

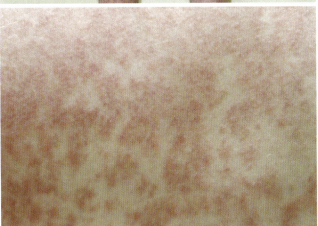

Fig. 20.2 Maculopapular exanthema. Infectious mononucleosis

20.2 Other Exanthemas

Table 20.2 Other diseases that may be exanthematous (lesions appear quickly but the rash is generally longer lasting)

Nature of lesions	Main causes
Papules and/or erythematous or erythematosquamous plaques	Cutaneous Kikuchi disease (face, often necrotic)
	Lymphomatoid papulosis
	Eruptive syringomas
	Eruptive xanthomas
	Erythema multiforme
	Exanthematous lichen
	Generalized granuloma annulare
	Gianotti-Crosti syndrome
	Pityriasis rosea of Gibert
	Grover's disease
	Guttate psoriasis
	Leukocytoclastic vasculitis
	Lichen nitidus (sometimes generalized and exanthematous)
	Lichen scrofulosorum and tuberculids
	Liebow's granulomatosis
	Lupus erythematosus
	Lymphoma, leukemia, histiocytosis
	Nephrogenic systemic fibrosis (formerly known as nephrogenic sclerosing dermopathy)
	Pityriasis lichenoides
	Prurigo
	Secondary syphilis
	Septicemia (specific cutaneous localization)
	Sweet syndrome
Vesicles and pustules	Acute generalized exanthematous pustulosis
	Coxsackie virus
	Grover's disease
	Neutrophilic dermatoses
	Pustular psoriasis
	Varicella (chicken pox)

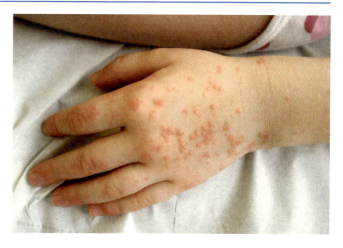

Fig. 20.4 Papular exanthema. Gianotti-Crosti syndrome. The rash occurs mostly on the extremities. It is a paraviral eruption, as several different viruses can produce this clinical picture

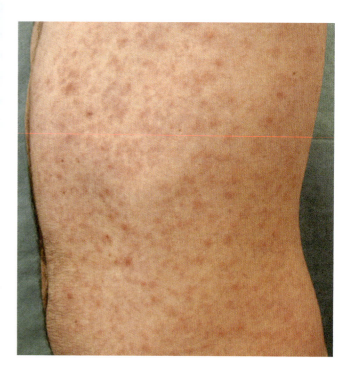

Fig. 20.5 Papular exanthema. Secondary syphilis. Such an appearance commands a serodiagnosis for syphilis

Papules

Diffuse papular eruptions may reveal septicemia (bacterial or fungal); this must be kept in mind especially in immunosuppressed individuals. Purpuric papulopustules must be considered as cutaneous localizations of septicemia until proven otherwise. Such lesions can also be seen during certain vasculitis such as Behçet's disease.

A secondary syphilis must not be overlooked while considering a papular eruption.

Histiocytosis and lymphomas/leukemias, as well as Liebow's disease and angioimmunoblastic lymphadenopathy, can all have eruptive manifestations. The diagnosis of eruptive xanthomas may be a medical emergency because of the potentially fatal complications of hypertriglyceridemia (pancreatitis, Zieve's syndrome)

Common

Pityriasis rosea of Gibert and psoriasis

Vesicles and Pustules

Pustules, especially purpuric ones, can uncover a septicemia (*gonococci*, *meningococci*).

A viral infection should also always be considered: herpes, VZV (varicella zoster virus), Coxsackie virus, smallpox, etc. Finally, some serious drug eruptions are pustular: AGEP, DRESS.

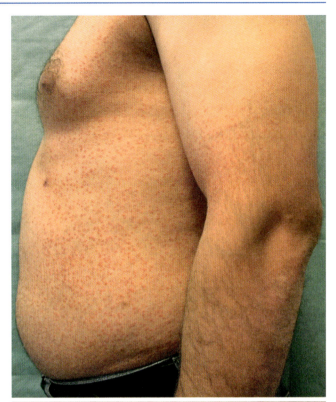

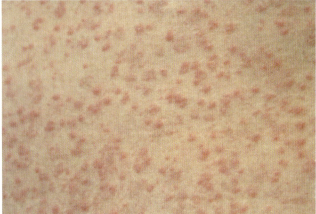

Fig. 20.6 Disseminated red papules. Disseminated granuloma annulare. These are dermal papules with no alteration of the skin surface. Granuloma annulare can sometimes occur in an eruptive way and can be generalized and only slightly annular or not at all

Erythroderma

21

The differential diagnosis of erythroderma (cf. Figs. 3.11, 14.28, and 14.29), which has numerous causes, can be difficult due to the fact that the clinical picture is the same regardless of the causative disorder. Hence the importance of history taking, especially regarding previous dermatoses (such as psoriasis or mycosis fungoides), as well as drugs taken. History of the disease must also be very precise; a localized onset with pruritus and oozing, preceding a secondary generalization, may, for example, suggest a secondarily generalized contact dermatitis.

Careful clinical examination sometimes allows identifying primary lesions that are characteristic of the initial dermatosis (e.g., typical papules of lichen planus). These lesions must be looked for and biopsied in order to establish diagnosis. Examination of the scalp and mucous membranes must not be omitted. Finally, clinicians should bear in mind that, regardless of the cause of erythroderma, this syndrome has consequences on the general health condition that can be life threatening. Consequently, some patients may need to be hospitalized in specialized dermatology departments.

Table 21.1 Main causes of an erythroderma

Age of onset	Main causes
Adult	Erythrodermic dermatoses:
	Dermatitis (contact, atopic, etc.)
	Seborrheic dermatitis (rare)
	Psoriasis
	Lichen (planus)
	Pemphigus foliaceous
	Pityriasis rubra pilaris
	Chronic actinic dermatitis
	Others: dermatomyositis, subacute cutaneous lupus erythematosus, bullous pemphigoid, etc.
	Drug-induced erythroderma
	Hematological disorders and cutaneous lymphoma:
	Mycosis fungoides, Sézary's syndrome
	Lymphomas, leukemias
	Erythrodermas of various causes:
	Infectious: bacterial (staphylococcal scalded skin syndrome or SSSS), fungal (candidiasis, trichophytosis, etc.), parasitic (scabies)
	HIV linked erythrodermas
	Graft-versus-host reaction
	Paraneoplastic
	Idiopathic
Newborn and infant	Atopic dermatitis
	Causes of adult erythrodermas
	Congenital and neonatal candidiasis
	Erythrodermic mastocytosis
	Graft-versus-host reaction (possibility of placental transfer)
	Ichthyoses: congenital ichthyosiform erythrodermas and Netherton syndrome
	Immune deficiencies (Omenn syndrome)
	Langerhans cell histiocytosis
	Metabolic disorders (carboxylase deficiency, EFA, etc.)
	Seborrheic dermatitis (Leiner-Moussous)
	Staphylococcal (SSSS and TSS)

TSS toxic shock syndrome, *EFA* essential fatty acids

D. Lipsker, *Clinical Examination and Differential Diagnosis of Skin Lesions*,
DOI 10.1007/978-2-8178-0411-8_21, © Springer-Verlag France 2013

Do Not Miss

An erythroderma may reveal a cancer or lymphoma and some infections can become erythrodermic: HIV infection, scabies, and candidiasis in the newborn.

Common

Drug eruption, generalized dermatitis, and psoriasis

Livedo

22

It is important to distinguish between the following:

- Livedo reticularis, a netlike erythema with fine, regular, and complete ("closed") meshes, which is more common and generally physiological.
- Livedo racemosa with large, sometimes broken meshes, which is always pathological and characteristic of Sneddon's syndrome, for example.
- Infiltrated, palpable livedo associated with sometimes purpuric papules, plaques, or nodules, mainly observed in vasculitis, such as polyarteritis nodosa (cf. Fig. 15.32).
- Purpuric livedo or retiform purpura which is indicative of a thrombotic vasculopathy involving the dermal vessels with muscular walls (cf. Figs. 14.13, 14.14, and 14.15); this type of livedo can be seen, for example, in disseminated intravascular coagulation or in catastrophic antiphospholipid antibody syndrome. The key significance of this livedo is discussed in Chap. 14.

Table 22.1 Main causes of livedo according to mechanism

Mechanisms	Main causes
Vasomotor disorder: mainly livedo reticularis	Disorders of the central nervous system: multiple sclerosis, encephalopathy, poliomyelitis, Parkinson's disease, stroke, traumatic brain trauma, etc.
	Drugs: amantadine, vasopressors, phenylbutazone, β-blockers
	Hypothyroidism, cushing syndrome, pellagra
	Low cardiac output (heart failure, shock)
	Physiological livedo of the newborn and *cutis marmorata telangiectatica congenita* (often racemosa)
	Pheochromocytoma, carcinoid (through the release of vasoactive substances)

(continued)

Embolisms: livedo racemosa and retiform purpura	Cholesterol embolisms (atheroembolism)
	Embolisms (including in association with auricular myxoma and endocarditis)
	Gas (air) embolisms (decompression sickness or caisson disease)
	Infectious embolisms (bacterial and viral)
	Intralymphatic histiocytosis (associated with rheumatoid arthritis)
	Malignant embolisms (intravascular lymphoma, visceral cancers)
	Nicolau's livedoid dermatitis (by accidental intra-arterial injection)
	Paradoxical embolisms via *foramen ovale*
Hyperviscosity: livedo racemosa	Blood hypercellularity: myeloproliferative disorder, leukemias
	Increased plasma viscosity: paraprotein, cold agglutinins, cryoglobulinemia, cryofibrinogenemia, antiphospholipid antibodies, etc.
	Pancreatitis
Thromboses: livedo racemosa and retiform purpura	APS, cryoglobulinemia
	Deficiency in coagulation proteins
	DIC
	Thrombotic microangiopathies (Moschcowitz syndrome, etc.)
Small artery disease (degenerative, metabolic, inflammatory, endoproliferative): livedo racemosa and/or infiltrated	Atheroma
	Hypertensive leg ulcer
	Livedoid vasculitis
	Nodular vasculitis
	Post-hypertensive vessel sclerosis
	Sneddon's syndrome
	Systemic vasculitis (PAN, granulomatosis with angiitis, etc.)
Crystal deposits: retiform purpura	Calciphylaxis
	Oxaluria, homocystinuria

CNS central nervous system, *CVA* cerebrovascular accident, *APS* antiphospholipid syndrome, *DIC* disseminated intravascular coagulation, *PAN* polyarteritis nodosa

Do Not Miss

Livedo racemosa and retiform purpura are cutaneous expressions of serious vascular diseases and they indicate endoluminal thrombosis or embolisms. For example, retiform purpura is one of the signs of purpura fulminans. An infiltrated livedo is the marker of a vasculitis.

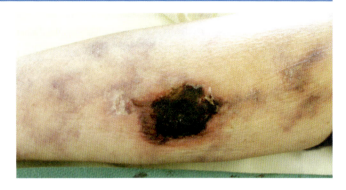

Fig. 22.3 Necrotizing livedo. Calciphylaxis

Common

Livedo reticularis, mostly physiological

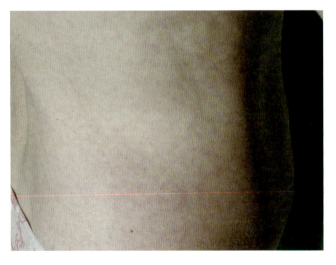

Fig. 22.1 Regular netlike erythema with fine and regular meshes. Physiological livedo

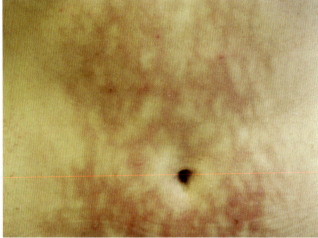

Fig. 22.4 Reticulate erythema (livedo) of the abdomen, with evolution towards pigmentary sequelae. Erythema ab igne

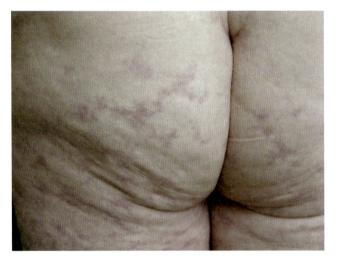

Fig. 22.2 Irregular mottled erythema in the pattern of large and sometimes broken meshes. Livedo racemosa

Purpura

23

There are several semiological variants of purpura, some of which have a diagnostic value:

- Stellate and retiform purpura (cf. Figs. 14.13, 14.14, 14.15, and 14.16): thrombosing vasculopathy
- Palpable (infiltrated) purpura (cf. Fig. 3.15): vasculitis
- Purpuric papulopustules (cf. Figs. 5.9, 14.20, and 12.52): septicemias, particularly caused by gonococci
- Perifollicular purpura: scurvy

- Ecchymotic purpura accompanied by bleeding (cf. Figs. 3.14, 14.18, and 14.19): disorders of primary hemostasis

Until proven otherwise, purpura should always be considered as a sign of a medical emergency, e.g., meningococcemia, endocarditis, and purpuras related to thrombocytopenia and/or disseminated intravascular coagulation. For teaching purposes, the causes of palpable purpuras are also illustrated in this chapter.

Table 23.1 Main causes of non-palpable purpura

Petechial lesion	Ecchymotic lesion (with or without petechiae)
Bacteremia and septicemia (particularly bacterial endocarditis)	Angioimmunoblastic lymphadenopathy
DIC (usually ecchymotic and gangrenous and/or retiform purpura)	Bateman's purpura (mechanical cause)
Infection with parvovirus B19 and other viruses	DIC (multiple causes) and particularly septicemia caused by infection with *meningococcus, pneumococcus, streptococcus, staphylococcus, Rickettsiae*, Gram-negative bacteria
Langerhans cell histiocytosis	Ehlers-Danlos syndrome
Paraproteinemia (particularly cryoglobulinemia)	Gardner-Diamond syndrome (causing painful ecchymoses)
Purpuric and pigmentary dermatitis	(Primary) amyloidosis
Purpuric granuloma annulare (exceptional)	Pseudo-hematoma: specific location in myeloid leukemia, cutaneous hematopoiesis, myeloproliferative or myelodysplastic syndrome, Langerhans cell histiocytosis, angiotropic lymphoma, metastases (e.g., melanoma), angiosarcoma, Kaposi's disease, tufted angioma
Black heel	Retiform purpura in thrombotic livedos (cf. Chap. 22)
Drug eruption	Anticoagulant therapy (overdosage, idiosyncratic and immune reaction)
Infections with *Rickettsiae*	Scurvy
Stasis (purpura due to hydrostatic pressure, particularly in the lower limbs)	Superficial and hemorrhagic pyoderma gangrenosum
Thrombopenia and disorders of primary hemostasis	Thrombopenia and disorders of primary hemostasis
	Trauma
	Vasculitis (large-vessel angiitis and granulomatous angiitis, PAN, etc.), generally palpable purpura

DIC disseminated intravascular coagulation, *PAN* polyarteritis nodosa

D. Lipsker, *Clinical Examination and Differential Diagnosis of Skin Lesions,*
DOI 10.1007/978-2-8178-0411-8_23, © Springer-Verlag France 2013

Table 23.2 Main causes of palpable purpura

Vasculitic lesions	Non-vasculitic lesions (pseudopurpura)
Bacteremia (more often non-palpable)	Angiokeratoma
Henoch-Schönlein purpura	Botryomycoma
Langerhans cell histiocytosis	Kaposi's disease
Leukocytoclastic vasculitis	Ruby spots
Paraproteinemia (often non-palpable)	
Rickettsiae, typhus, etc.	

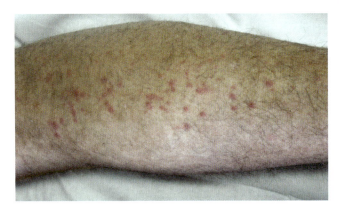

Fig. 23.1 Purpuric papules. Cryoglobulinemia (related to hepatitis C viral infection)

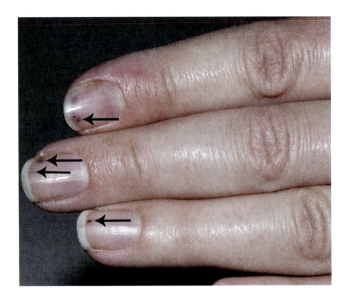

Fig. 23.2 Fine linear purpura affecting the nail bed. Flame-shaped hemorrhages (*arrows*). Distal lesions are common in manual workers. Proximal and/or multiple lesions may reflect a thrombosing vasculopathy that can appear in various contexts: infectious endocarditis, non-septic emboli (e.g., auricular myxoma), antiphospholipid antibody syndrome, hypereosinophilic syndrome, etc

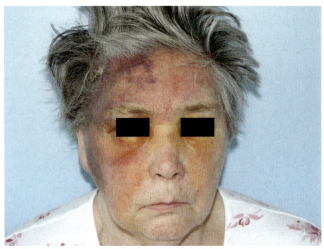

Fig. 23.3 Pseudo-ecchymosis. Angiosarcoma of the head

Do Not Miss

Purpura (even in the petechial form) can be the first sign of a serious infection such as meningococcemia or endocarditis. It can also be the manifestation of a disorder of primary hemostasis, for example, thrombopenia, in which case it is often associated with bleeding. Therefore, it commands a complete blood count, including platelets, as well as a coagulation profile. Finally, thrombosing vasculopathies, among which are life-threatening emergencies such as catastrophic antiphospholipid antibody syndrome or DIC, often manifest as stellate purpuric macules and/or purpuric livedo (retiform purpura). Palpable purpura is a sign of vasculitis.

Common

Stasis purpura, senile purpura (dermatoporosis), and many dermatoses can become purpuric in patients receiving anticoagulants.

Telangiectases

There are several semiological variants of telangiectases, some of which have a diagnostic value:

- Arborising pattern (cf. Fig. 3.12a).
- Stellate (cf. Fig. 3.12a).
- Rectangular macules (cf. Fig. 15.27): common in sclerodermas.
- Papular (cf. Fig. 15.94): common in Rendu-Osler disease; to be distinguished from ruby spots.
- Papular and keratotic: angiokeratomas; when multiple and located in the underwear area, they command the search for Fabry disease (cf. Fig. 15.96).
- Periungual or gingival, also known as "mega-capillaries" (cf. Fig. 15.21) and highly suggestive of a connective tissue disease, particularly dermatopolymyositis and scleroderma.

- Associated with other lesions; present among lesions of poikiloderma or of the pearly border of basal cell carcinoma.

Certain telangiectases are the dermatologic manifestation of systemic diseases such as intravascular lymphoma or POEMS syndrome (polyneuropathy, organomegaly, endocrinopathy, monoclonal component, skin lesion). In patients with intravascular lymphoma, the biopsy of a telangiectasia allows to establish diagnosis, due to the fact that there is a proliferation of malignant lymphocytes that are usually easily observable within the dermal vessels. In the absence of a cutaneous lesion, the diagnosis of intravascular lymphoma which often affects the central nervous system and can mimic vasculitis and can be very difficult to establish.

Table 24.1 Main causes of telangiectases

Type of lesions	Main causes	
Acquired telangiectases	Not affecting the visceral organs (purely cutaneous forms)	*Localized*:
		Face: rosacea, following steroid therapy
		Idiopathic spider angiomas
		Senile angiomas (ruby spots or cherry angiomas)
		Lower limbs: circulatory disorders (chronic venous stasis)
		Telangiectases in purpuric dermatitis (Majocchi disease)
		Idiopathic generalized essential telangiectases (onset)
		Postlesional: radiodermatitis, basal cell carcinoma
		On a dermatome[a]: unilateral nevoid telangiectases[b]
		Ubiquitous and/or generalized:
		Senile skin, cutaneous atrophy following corticosteroid therapy
		Idiopathic generalized essential telangiectases
		Cutaneous collagenous vasculopathy
		Reticulate and telangiectatic erythema
		Erythema ab igne
	Associated to a disease or a general cause	Acquired poikilodermic disorders (mycosis fungoides, poikilodermatomyositis, subacute lupus erythematosus, chronic lichenoid drug eruption, chronic GVHR, POEMS syndrome)
		Carcinoid, polycythemia vera, mastocytoses
		Cirrhosis, liver cancer
		Connective tissue disorders: CREST syndrome, diffuse systemic sclerosis
		Fabry disease
		Intravascular lymphoma
		POEMS syndrome
		Pregnancy
		Pulmonary arterial hypertension, thoracic tumors, auricular myxoma
		Telangiectatic mastocytosis
		Toxic substances and drugs: aluminum, calcium channel blockers
		Viral Infections: HIV, echovirus, HVC
Congenital or hereditary telangiectases[c]		Ataxia-telangiectasia
		Congenital poikilodermas
		Cutis marmorata telangiectatica congenita
		Fabry disease and other metabolic overload diseases
		Focal dermal hypoplasia
		Hereditary hemorrhagic telangiectases, Rendu-Osler disease
		Hereditary benign telangiectases
		Rombo syndrome
		Serpiginous angioma
		Unilateral nevoid telangiectases (congenital forms)
		Xeroderma pigmentosum

CREST subcutaneous calcinosis, Raynaud's syndrome, esophageal involvement, sclerodactylia and telangiectases, *HIV* human immunodeficiency virus, *VHC* hepatitis C virus, *POEMS* polyneuropathy, organomegaly, endocrinopathy, monoclonal component, skin lesion, *GVHR* graft-versus-host reaction

[a]Not always strict

[b]Sometimes associated with traumas or ipsilateral bone malformations

[c]May seem acquired

Do Not Miss

Telangiectases may reveal intravascular lymphoma, POEMS syndrome, Fabry disease, ataxia-telangiectasia, or Rendu-Osler disease. Multiple telangiectases with numerous spider nevus in the upper half of the body are classically found in cirrhosis; telangiectases are also present in certain connective tissue diseases (Sharp syndrome, systemic sclerosis) and in a particular clinical form of mastocytosis. They can also be seen in thoracic tumors, in PAH (pulmonary arterial hypertension), auricular myxoma, and in certain viral infections (HIV, HCV, echovirus).

Common

Physiological, pregnancy and aging. Venous insufficiency. Rosacea. Following steroid therapy. Ruby spots (or cherry angioma) and spider nevus.

Yellow, Orange, and Green Macules

25

These lesions are rare but quite visible because of their bright color. They have partly been addressed in the chapter dealing with hyperpigmented lesions.

Lesions may be localized or diffused. In the presence of diffused lesions, associated involvement of the mucous and/or conjunctival membranes must be searched.

The *yellow* color can be the result of cutaneous deposits of fat, bile salts, drugs or toxic substances, and carotene; it can also be the consequence of the production of intradermal granulomas and/or alteration of the elastic tissue or a regressing hematoma.

A real *orange* color is very rare. It is found in juvenile xanthogranulomas. Amyloidosis and PRP (pityriasis rubra pilaris) may confer to the skin a diffuse orange appearance.

The *green* color can be of toxic origin (i.e., exogenous hair coloration by copper-chlorine water), metabolic (porphyrias, tyrosyluria), or correspond to a cutaneous location of hematopoietic cells (chloroma) or to a regressing hematoma.

Box 25.1 Main Causes of Yellow Lesions

Amyloidosis
Carotenoid pigmentation
Fordyce nodule (on mucosa)
Icterus (jaundice)
Necrobiosis lipoidica
Palmoplantar keratoderma
Pseudoxanthoma elasticum
Solar elastosis
Xanthomas

D. Lipsker, *Clinical Examination and Differential Diagnosis of Skin Lesions*,
DOI 10.1007/978-2-8178-0411-8_25, © Springer-Verlag France 2013

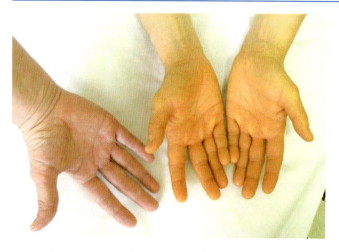

Fig. 25.1 Yellow hands (xanthoderma). Carotenoid pigmentation. It usually has a dietary cause (excessive consumption of carrots, spinach, or pumpkins) and often occurs in patients with anorexia nervosa. Carotenoid pigmentation can sometimes reveal a hyperlipemia, a para-proteinemia, or a congenital anomaly in carotenoid metabolism

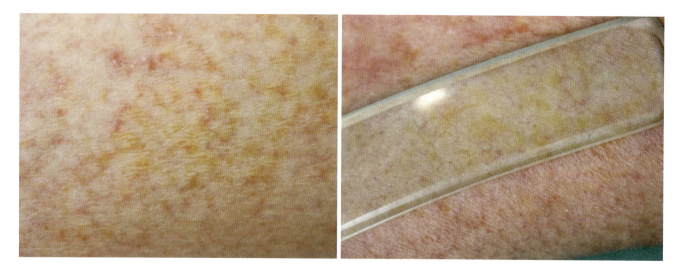

Fig. 25.2 Yellow xanthodermic macules on a slightly scaly, erythematous, and telangiectatic background. Mycosis fungoides. Note that the yellow coloration becomes more visible on diascopy

Dermo-epidermal Atrophy, Lipoatrophy, and Lipodystrophy

26.1 Dermo-epidermal Atrophy
(cf. Figs. 2.4, 3.16, 6.5, and 6.8)

Some atrophic lesions are more visible than palpable and are thus classified as macules. Among atrophic dermatoses, some are exclusively atrophic (e.g., superficial and/or mid-dermal elastolysis), while in others, atrophy is only part of the various existing primary lesions. This is particularly the case in poikiloderma (addressed in Chap. 27), where atrophy is associated with telangiectases and reticulate pigmentary changes.

Cutaneous atrophy is one of the signs of skin aging (cf. Figs. 12.61, 12.62, and 12.63). Cutaneous atrophy can be important in patients with rheumatoid arthritis, endogenous or iatrogenic hypercorticism, or who are being treated with hydroxyurea. Cutaneous atrophy is associated with other dermatological lesions in connective tissue diseases, such as lupus erythematosus and dermatomyositis, infectious diseases (e.g., Lyme borreliosis and syphilis), certain immune deficiencies (e.g., TAP deficiency: transporter associated with antigen processing), and cutaneous T-cell lymphoma.

Causes of lipoatrophy are presented in Table 26.1.

Table 26.1 Main causes of dermal and epidermal atrophy

Acquired dermal and epidermal atrophy	Atrophic dermatoses
Aging	Acrodermatitis chronica atrophicans
Drug intake (steroids, hydroxyurea)	Atrophic pigmented dermatofibrosarcoma
Idiopathic atrophoderma	Atrophic and ulcerating sarcoidosis
Rheumatoid arthritis	Congenital atrophy (aplasia cutis, etc.)
	Dermatomyositis
	Discoid lupus erythematosus
	Elastolytic giant cell granuloma
	Granuloma annulare
	Hemifacial atrophy (Parry-Romberg syndrome)
	Lichen planus
	Lichen sclerosus
	Livedoid vasculopathy (atrophie blanche)
	Lupus miliaris disseminatus faciei
	Lupus vulgaris
	Medallion-like dermal dendrocyte hamartoma (plaque-like CD34-positive dermal fibroma)
	Mycosis fungoides (chalazodermic lymphoma and poikiloderma vasculare atrophicans)
	Necrobiosis lipoidica
	Neoplastic alopecia
	O'Brien's actinic granuloma
	Poikiloderma and all its related causes
	Porokeratosis
	Scarring sequelae of various dermatoses (acne, etc.)
	Scleroatrophic syndrome of Huriez
	Superficial and/or mid-dermal elastolysis
	Systemic sclerosis
	TAP deficiency
	Vermiculate atrophoderma

TAP transporter associated with antigen processing

D. Lipsker, *Clinical Examination and Differential Diagnosis of Skin Lesions*, DOI 10.1007/978-2-8178-0411-8_26, © Springer-Verlag France 2013

Do Not Miss
Certain cutaneous T-cell lymphomas and certain skin cancers evolve towards atrophy, as do some metastases.

Common
Skin aging and dermatoporosis.

26.2   Lipoatrophy and Lipodystrophy

Lipoatrophy causes a visible, often cup-shaped, depression of the skin (cf. Fig. 6.10). It can be localized, regional (limbs), or diffuse. It can be secondary to inflammation of the subcutis, in which case it is a sequela of panniculitis. When not preceded by inflammation, it is a primary lipoatrophy or lipodystrophy. These two situations are not always easy to differentiate. For example, in lupus erythematosus, both situations have been reported (i.e., primary lipoatrophy and sequelae of lupus panniculitis). In most instances, lipoatrophies are secondary disorders, occurring after injections or inflammatory diseases involving the subcutis. A lipoatrophy can be the manifestation of a systemic disease, for example, in POEMS syndrome, dermatopolymyositis, lupus erythematosus, various endocrinopathies, and HIV infection treated with protease inhibitors. When it is the initial manifestation of lupus erythematosus, for example, diagnosis can be difficult. Finally, there are hereditary diseases in which lipoatrophy can be prominent, among which are laminopathies.

Table 26.2   Main causes of lipoatrophies and lipodystrophies

Localized	Acquired partial lipodystrophy (Barraquer-Simons syndrome) (face)
	Acromegaly, thyroid dysfunction (generalized lipodystrophies)
	Annular lipoatrophy
	Cushing syndrome (limbs)
	Deep morphea and hemifacial atrophy (Parry-Romberg syndrome)
	Diabetes
	Familial partial lipodystrophy (Köbberling-Dunnigan syndrome) (limbs ± trunk)
	HIV treated with HIV-protease inhibitors (face and limbs) or HIV-nucleoside reverse transcriptase inhibitors
	Lipodystrophia centrifugalis abdominalis infantilis
	Subcutaneous lymphoma
	Injection-induced (corticoids, insulin, iron, vaccines, penicillin G, growth hormone, etc.)
	Lupus erythematosus
	POEMS syndrome
	Postinflammatory sequela
	Rheumatoid arthritis
	Semicircular lipoatrophy
	Tumors of the anterior pituitary gland (phenotype close to the Barraquer-Simons syndrome)
Generalized	Acquired generalized lipodystrophy (or Lawrence syndrome)
	Congenital generalized lipodystrophy (or Berardinelli-Seip syndrome)
In the newborn	AREDYLD syndrome
	Cockayne syndrome
	Leprechaunism (lipodystrophy, insulin resistance, acanthosis nigricans, hirsutism)
	Progeria-like
	SHORT syndrome

POEMS polyneuropathy, organomegaly, endocrinopathy, monoclonal component, skin lesion, *HIV* human immunodeficiency virus, *AREDYLD* acral renal ectodermal dysplasia lipoatrophic diabetes, *SHORT* short stature, hyperextensibility of joints, ocular depression, Rieger or ocular and dental anomaly, teething delay

Do Not Miss
HIV infection, endocrinopathies, and systemic diseases such as lupus erythematosus.

Common
Postinjection and postinflammatory.

Poikiloderma must be distinguished from reticulate pigmentary disorders without atrophy or telangiectases and from non-atrophic telangiectatic dermatoses. It can be localized or diffuse, and associated or not with other primary lesions, which would then contribute to diagnosis. Hereditary poikilodermas appearing in childhood are usually differentiated from acquired adult forms. However, certain hereditary diseases do not become poikilodermic until adulthood, whereas certain acquired poikilodermic diseases can appear in early childhood.

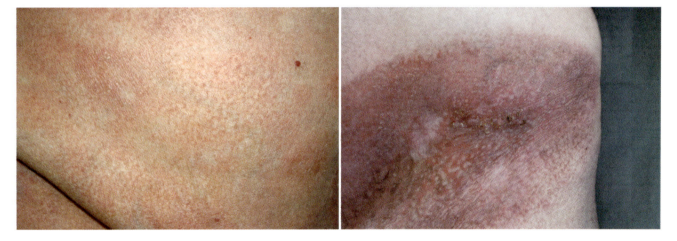

Fig. 27.1 Poikiloderma. Mycosis fungoides

D. Lipsker, *Clinical Examination and Differential Diagnosis of Skin Lesions*,
DOI 10.1007/978-2-8178-0411-8_27, © Springer-Verlag France 2013

Table 27.1 Main causes of poikilodermas

Hereditary or congenital poikilodermas	Acquired poikiloderma
Familial spastic paraplegia with neuropathy and poikiloderma	Chronic graft-versus-host reaction
Fanconi's (pernicious) anemia	Dermatomyositis
Fat overload related diseases	Lichen planus
Imerslund-Grasbeck syndrome	Lupus erythematosus (subacute)
Kindler syndrome	Macular amyloidosis
Mendes da Costa syndrome	Mycosis fungoides
PARC syndrome	Poikiloderma of Civatte
Poikiloderma with tendon retraction, hyperhidrosis and pulmonary fibrosis	Radiodermatitis and skin response to chronic exposure to cold or hot temperatures
Poikiloderma with neutropenia (Clericuzio type)	Systemic sclerosis (rarely)
Rothmund-Thomson syndrome	Treatment with hydroxyurea
Scleroatrophic syndrome of Huriez	
Weary syndrome	
Werner syndrome	
Xeroderma pigmentosum	
Zinsser-Cole-Engman syndrome	

PARC poikiloderma, alopecia, retrognathism, and cleft palate

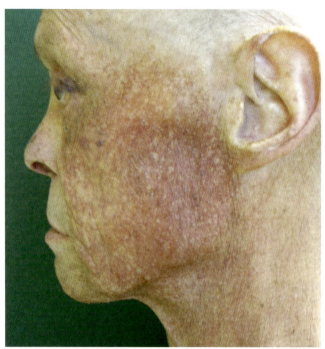

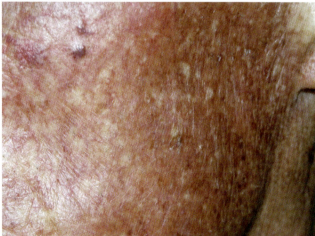

Fig. 27.2 Congenital autosomal dominant poikiloderma with tendon retraction. Alopecia is not related to this syndrome; it was the consequence of chemotherapy administered for pancreatic carcinoma

Do Not Miss

Acquired poikiloderma can be a sign of cutaneous T-cell lymphoma, dermatomyositis, lupus erythematosus, graft-versus-host disease, and Zinsser-Cole-Engman syndrome of late onset. Several inherited diseases can manifest as poikiloderma that appears during childhood.

Common

Poikiloderma of Civatte.

Vesicles and Bullae

28

Some disorders can be either vesicular or bullous. Hence, the causes of these two types of primary lesions are addressed together.

A vesicle must not be confused with a molluscum contagiosum, a milia seed, or a cystic lymphangioma.

Vesicles are mainly caused by infectious diseases (i.e., viral and parasitic infections), dermatitis, and autoimmune bullous dermatoses such as dermatitis herpetiformis and linear IgA dermatosis. In viral diseases such as infections with *Herpesviridae*, lesions are often umbilicated, i.e., with a central depression or dell, and can be pruritic, but without oozing. Viral vesicles usually have a particular gray color, especially in initial stages. However, in dermatitis, lesions are always pruritic and oozing. Certain systemic diseases may rarely manifest as vesicles, which are then accompanied by other primary lesions, e.g., subacute cutaneous lupus erythematosus or acrodermatitis enteropathica.

Bullae resulting from intraepidermal fragility break easily. They then evolve towards more or less superficial and round erosions, lined by a collarette which allows retrospective diagnosis.

Common causes of bullae are an overly elevated hydrostatic pressure (e.g., an edema flare-up in the lower limbs), mechanical stress (e.g., foot blisters), infections (i.e., impetigo), hypersensitivities (i.e., bullous dermatitis, dyshidrosis, and drug eruptions), and pemphigoid in patients over 65. However, several diseases may have a usual or unusual bullous manifestation, which is then generally associated with other cutaneous signs, such as in infectious bullous cellulitis or in bullous morphea.

Table 28.1 Main causes of vesicles and bullae

Diseases that are mainly vesicular	Diseases that are mainly bullous
Autoimmune dermatoses	*Autoimmune dermatoses*
Dermatitis herpetiformis	Acquired bullous epidermolysis bullosa
Linear IgA dermatosis.	Autoimmune and paraneoplastic pemphigus
Dermatitis and dyshidrosis	Bullous disease associated with monoclonal IgM
Infections	Bullous forms of vasculitis (usually hemorrhagic) and of thromboses (DIC)
Prurigo strophulus	Bullous lupus erythematosus
Scabies	Bullous pemphigoid
Vesicular dermatophytosis	Dermatitis herpetiformis (mostly vesicular)
Virus infections: herpes, zoster, Coxsackie virus, vaccine	Linear IgA dermatosis
Grover's disease	Other rare autoimmune bullous diseases
Tumors	*Congenital or hereditary*
Vesicular mycosis fungoides	Congenital bullous ichtyosiform erythroderma
Transient myeloproliferative syndrome of the newborn	Congenital poikiloderma with bulla formation
Inflammatory dermatoses	Darier's disease
Bullous acrodermatitis enteropathica (and related disorders)	Hailey-Hailey disease
Pityriasis lichenoides (usually papular)	Hereditary epidermolysis bullosa
Vesicobullous lichen planus	Incontinentia pigmenti

(continued)

D. Lipsker, *Clinical Examination and Differential Diagnosis of Skin Lesions*,
DOI 10.1007/978-2-8178-0411-8_28, © Springer-Verlag France 2013

Table 28.1 (continued)

Diseases that are mainly vesicular	Diseases that are mainly bullous
Vesicular subacute lupus erythematosus	*Drug eruptions*
Miscellaneous	Bullous fixed drug eruption
Hidrocystoma (pseudovesicle)	Lyell's syndrome, Stevens-Johnson syndrome
Incontinentia pigmenti	Phototoxicity
Mercury intoxication (mostly on palms)	*External agents (physical, chemical, etc.)*
	Burns related to heat, sun (UV), radiations, chemicals, etc.
	Factitial dermatitis
	Frictional bulla
	Insect bite
	Phytophotodermatitis
	Polymorphous light eruption
	Infections
	Arbovirus infections (Chikungunya)
	Bullous ecthyma gangrenosum due to *Pseudomonas aeruginosa* and septicemia caused by other Gram (−) bacilli
	Bullous erysipelas and bullous cellulitis
	Bullous impetigo
	Congenital syphilis
	Erysipeloid
	Severe cellulitis and necrotizing fasciitis
	Staphylococcal scalded skin syndrome
	Inflammatory diseases and miscellaneous
	Acrodermatitis enteropathica
	Bullae caused by hydrostatic pressure
	Bullous forms of various dermatoses: dermatitis, urticaria, Sweet syndrome lichen planus, mastocytosis etc.
	Bullous mastocytosis
	Bullous paraneoplastic acrokeratosis (or Bazex syndrome)
	Erythema multiforme (bullous)
	Grover's disease (usually papules and papulopustules)
	Necrolytic migratory erythema (i.e., glucagonoma syndrome)
	Subcorneal pustulosis
	Systemic sclerosis and bullous morphea
	Toxic coma-associated bullosis
	Metabolic and overload diseases
	Bullous amyloidosis
	Bullosis diabeticorum
	Pellagra
	Porphyria (cutanea tarda, erythropoietic, etc.)
	Pseudo-porphyria (in patients undergoing dialysis, etc.)

Vesicles

In a patient with a vesicular eruption, consider the possibility of a viral infection (herpes, VZV, Coxsackie virus, smallpox), especially when vesicles are gray and evolve towards umbilication.

Common

Dermatitis and dyshidrosis, virus infection, dermatophytosis, and scabies.

Bullae

Widespread bullae of acute onset and/or extensive skin detachment can be seen in drug-induced Lyell's syndrome, bullous (super)acute lupus erythematosus, linear IgA dermatosis (particularly induced by vancomycin), paraneoplastic pemphigus, bullous and generalized fixed drug eruption, and graft-versus-host reaction. Bullous forms of vasculitides, thromboses and bullous acrokeratosis paraneoplastica (or Bazex syndrome), should not be overlooked.

A single bulla, usually hemorrhagic, can be observed at sites of inflammation such as an erysipela or a necrotizing fasciitis.

In septicemias caused by *Pseudomonas aeruginosa* bacteria, ecthyma gangrenosum usually appears as a hemorrhagic bullous plaque.

Finally, palmoplantar neonatal bullae are highly suggestive of congenital syphilis.

Common

External factors (friction, burn), as well as hydrostatic factors, pemphigoid, impetigo, and prurigo strophulus.

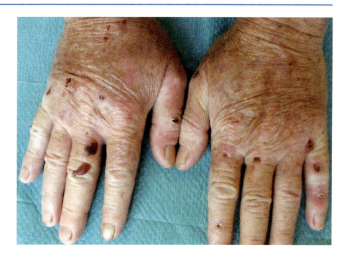

Fig. 28.2 Hemorrhagic bullae. Porphyria cutanea tarda. Also note the scars and crusts

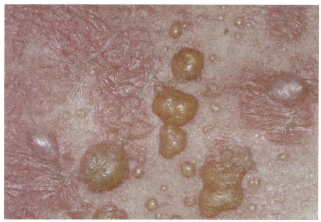

Fig. 28.3 Flaccid bullae. Pemphigus

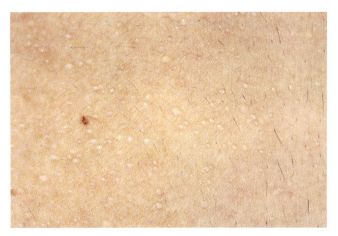

Fig. 28.1 Vesicle. Sweat duct milia. Multiple, tense lesions containing a translucent liquid. These lesions can appear with extreme heat and profuse sweating

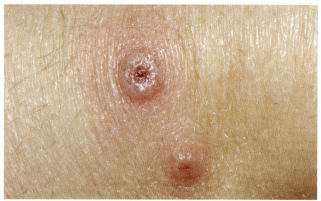

Fig. 28.4 Umbilicated bulla. Pyoderma gangrenosum. Umbilication is strongly suggestive of a viral cause. However, such lesions can also be seen in pyoderma gangrenosum and certain ANCA+, vasculitides, which raises the question of the role of *Herpesviridae* viruses in triggering flare-ups, at least of a cutaneous nature

Pustules

29

Pustules are either septic or aseptic; hence, microbiological examination of their content should always be performed. Bacteriological, mycological, and virological examinations are almost always recommended. Although pustules are caused by highly common and prevalent diseases such as acne, rosacea, and folliculitis, it is important to remember that a pustule can also be the primary lesion in certain severe illnesses requiring emergency treatment, such as septicemia and endocarditis. Finally, aseptic pustules can be the dermatological manifestation of many inflammatory diseases such as inflammatory bowel disease or lupus erythematosus.

Table 29.1 Main causes of pustules

Type[a]	Main causes
Septic pustule, usually follicular	Acne and induced acne (chlorine, drugs, tar, mineral oil)
	Cephalic pustulosis caused by infection with *Malassezia* (sympodialis)
	Folliculitis (caused by bacterial, fungal, and viral infections)
	Mycotic pustules (candidiasis, trichophytosis)
	Pyodermas
	Septicemias (chronic gonococcemia, meningococcemia, staphylococcemia, endocarditis, Listeria, Gram-bacteria, etc.)
	Superinfected vesicle
	Typical and atypical mycobacterial infections
	Viral pustules (herpes, orf, etc.)

Table 29.1 (continued)

Type	Main causes
Aseptic pustule, usually non-follicular	Circumoral dermatitis
	Eosinophilic folliculitis (Ofuji syndrome)
	Infantile acropustulosis
	Pustular granuloma annulare
	Toxic erythema of the newborn
	Acute generalized exanthematous pustulosis and pustular drug eruptions (follicular and non-follicular) as well as mercury exanthem
	Erosive pustulosis of the legs and scalp
	Halogenodermas
	Hidradenitis suppurativa (also called acne inverse or "Verneuil's disease" in the French terminology)
	Impetigo herpetiformis
	Neonatal eosinophilic pustulosis
	Palmoplantar pustuloses (psoriasis, reactive arthritis, recurrent vesicular acropustulosis, pustular dyshidrosis, etc.)
	Pemphigus vegetans
	Pustular psoriasis
	Pustulosis associated with systemic diseases (myeloma, blind loop syndrome, Crohn's disease, ulcerative colitis, Behçet's disease, amicrobial pustulosis associated with autoimmune diseases, etc.)
	Rosacea and pyoderma faciale
	Subcorneal pustulosis of Sneddon-Wilkinson and IgA pemphigus
	Transient myeloproliferative disorder in newborns
	Transient neonatal pustular melanosis
Pustular alopecia	Cheloid acne
	Dissecting cellulitis of the scalp
	Erosive pustulosis of the scalp
	Folliculitis decalvans
	Folliculocentric Langerhans cell histiocytosis
	Tinea

[a]A pustule should not be confused with milia seed, keratosis pilaris or miliaria crystallina

D. Lipsker, *Clinical Examination and Differential Diagnosis of Skin Lesions*, DOI 10.1007/978-2-8178-0411-8_29, © Springer-Verlag France 2013

Do Not Miss

Pustules, particularly purpuric ones, can uncover a septicemia (caused by infection with *Gonococci, Meningococci, Listeria, Staphylococcus,* and *Gram-bacteria*) or an endocarditis. Mycobacterial infections can be pustular (follicular). Pustules of the palms and soles are common in reactive arthritis.

Herpes and congenital candidiasis should always be suspected in the newborn. In general, the possibility of a viral infection should always be raised: herpes, VZV, Coxsackie virus, smallpox, etc.

The diagnoses of an IgA pemphigus, a subcorneal pustulosis of Sneddon-Wilkinson, and pustuloses encountered in systemic diseases (such as myeloma, CIBD, lupus erythematosus, SAPHO) should be considered in the presence of mostly non-follicular aseptic pustules.

Finally, certain severe drug eruptions are pustular: AGEP, DRESS.

Common

Acne and folliculitis (caused by infection with *Staphylococcus* and *Pityrosporum*), rosacea, pustules encountered in mycoses, and viral infections. Pustular drug eruptions and pustular psoriasis are not rare.

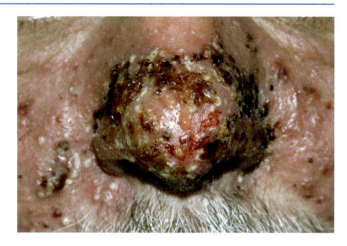

Fig. 29.1 Pustules, erosions and crusts. Cutaneous reaction after anti-EGFR treatment

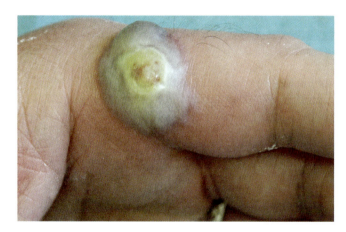

Fig. 29.2 Pustule caused by a viral infection. Orf

Palpable Lesions: Overview

30

Palpable lesions may be solid or contain fluid; in the latter case, one must refer to the chapter dedicated to fluid-filled lesions (vesicles, bullae, or pustules, in Chaps. 5, 28, and 29).

Solid lesions are categorized according to shape and size. On white skin, it is convenient to differentiate solid lesions according to their color and to the presence of potential alterations of their surfaces, as is done with macules. Papules, plaques, and nodules have the same causes and will therefore be addressed together. Deep-seated nodules indicate an involvement of either the fatty lobules or the inter-adipose septa or the cutaneous vessels lined with muscular walls. Palpable lesions bearing surface alterations such as scaly erythematous lesions, and necrotic lesions are discussed later (Chap. 39). The causes of facial, acral, and periarticular papules are addressed in Chap. 37. The causes of keratodermas are recalled in Chap. 38, as this situation is often encountered in medical practice.

30.1 Single Lesions

Single lesions must first and foremost be suspected as being tumoral, benign, or malignant. An evolving lesion, which is heterogeneous, irregular, asymmetrical, or ulcerated, must be considered as malignant, particularly if it is pigmented. A dermal or deeper-seated nodule, especially when hard, must raise the possibility of a metastasis. Certain tumoral lesions have a characteristic clinical appearance (cylindroma, seborrheic keratosis, nodular basal cell carcinoma, etc.). Certain tumors are *painful*: eccrine spiradenoma, tricho- and angioleiomyoma, angiolipoma, neuroma, neurilemmoma (or schwannoma), glomus tumor, certain pilomatricomas, painful piezogenic papules, and painful nodule of the ear are the most typical. Numerous other palpable lesions can be painful (e.g., abscesses, erythema nodosum, granuloma annulare of the extremities). Biopsy provides the final ruling for any skin tumor which has not been clinically identified.

30.2 Multiple Lesions

Multiple palpable lesions can also be related to skin tumors or cysts. For example, they can be seborrheic keratoses or nevi, which are extremely common lesions. Other lesions can appear in the context of a genetic syndrome that causes a predisposition for developing multiple skin tumors, such as trichoepitheliomas, cylindromas, and eccrine spiradenomas in Brooke-Spiegler syndrome. Some cutaneous tumors may be the cutaneous marker of a predisposition for visceral cancers (e.g., trichilemmomas in Cowden syndrome). Other causes must also be suspected, i.e., inflammatory, infectious, metabolic, and overload diseases, as well as blood disorders. As such, amyloidosis, mucinoses, and Waldenström's disease, as well as sarcoidosis and fibroblastic rheumatism, can manifest as cutaneous papules. A biopsy must be interpreted by an experienced dermatopathologist aware of the clinical context, as special staining techniques may be required to reveal the presence of substances such as amyloid. Classical signs of inflammation, redness, warmth, edema, and pain, clearly direct towards inflammatory and infectious diseases. Some inflammatory dermatoses such as lichen planus are sometimes sufficiently characteristic to be identified clinically.

Do Not Miss

When dealing with purpura, even if non-palpable, always consider first a severe infection such as meningitis, acute, subacute and chronic meningococcemia, endocarditis, rickettsiosis, and other septicemias. Eliminate a DIC and other hematological causes.

Papules

Diffuse papular eruptions may reveal septicemia (either bacterial or fungal); this must be kept in mind particularly

D. Lipsker, *Clinical Examination and Differential Diagnosis of Skin Lesions*, DOI 10.1007/978-2-8178-0411-8_30, © Springer-Verlag France 2013

in immunosuppressed individuals. Purpuric papulopustules must be considered as cutaneous localizations of septicemia, until proven otherwise. This type of lesions can also be seen in certain vasculitides such as Behçet's disease.

While considering a papular eruption, a secondary syphilis must not be overlooked.

Histiocytosis and lymphomas/leukemias can have eruptive manifestations.

Due to the potentially fatal complications of hyperlipidemia (pancreatitis, Zieve's syndrome), the proper diagnosis of eruptive xanthomas is a medical emergency.

Plaques

Edematous, pruritic, and evanescent plaques are characteristic of urticaria. If the urticaria occurs in the course of a "true" anaphylaxis, it is often preceded by palmoplantar pruritus and is accompanied by respiratory signs (such as dyspnea and wheezing), digestive signs (abdominal pain, nausea, and diarrhea), and a drop in blood pressure.

Ulcerative and necrotizing plaques are observed in Gram (–) septicemias and particularly septicemias caused by *Pseudomonas aeruginosa* bacilli (e.g., ecthyma gangrenosum).

A plaque-type eruption can indicate lupus erythematosus, erythema multiforme, vasculitis, and neutrophilic dermatosis.

Deep-seated inflammatory nodules (or "nouures" in the French terminology) may exceptionally reveal an acute meningococcemia or a systemic bacterial infection (such as brucellosis and Q fever). Other infectious causes must always be considered, whether bacterial (namely, mycobacterial infections) or fungal. Other potentially severe causes are nodular fat necrosis associated with pancreatic disease, cytophagic histiocytic panniculitis, Weber-Christian panniculitis, and systemic vasculitides.

Nodule

Irrespective of associated signs, the clinician should always suspect the diagnosis of metastasis or of cutaneous localization of lymphoma/leukemia in patients with one or more nodules, particularly if the nodules are indurated. A sporotrichoid alignment suggests an infection (mycobacterial infection, leishmaniasis, and sporotrichosis).

Generally, a single, solid, palpable lesion is most of the time a tumor: other semiological characteristics (such as regularity, symmetry, color, borders, size) will determine whether an excision or a biopsy is indicated.

Common

A single, solid, palpable lesion is usually a tumor (whether epithelial, melanocytic, fibrocytic, vascular, nervous, adipocytic, etc.).

Otherwise, many common disorders can manifest as a palpable lesion, such as warts, insect bites, folliculitis, cysts, acne, and rosacea.

Skin-Colored Palpable Lesions

31

Table 31.1 Main causes of palpable solid lesions of the same color as normal skin, with no alteration of the skin surface

Melanocytic and non-melanocytic nevi, malformations, and tumors	Atypical fibroxanthoma
	Chondrodermatitis nodularis helicis[a]
	Cysts (i.e., epidermoid, trichilemmal, dermoid)
	Epithelial and adnexal tumors: early-stage skin cancers (particularly basal cell carcinoma), fibroepithelioma of Pinkus (or premalignant fibroepithelial tumors of Pinkus), benign and malignant adnexal tumors[a], dermatofibrosarcoma, etc.
	Fibromas, connective tissue hamartomas, sarcomas, and other tumors of the connective tissue
	Glomus tumor
	Lipomatous: lipoma, angiolipoma, nodulocystic lipodystrophy
	Melanocytic: achromic melanoma, achromic nevus
	Metastasis (especially nodule)
	Nerve tumor: neurofibroma, neuroma and other nerve tumors
	Nodular fasciitis
	Rhinophyma
	Scar (hypertrophic, cheloid)
	Skin tag
Overload diseases	Acral mucinosis
	Lipoid proteinosis (palpebral)
	Macroglobulinodermia (in patients with Waldenström's disease)
	Papular amyloidosis
	Tophus, calcinosis and osteoma cutis
Infections	Molluscum contagiosum
	Warts (flat and genital)[a]
Granulomatous and systemic diseases	Eosinophilic granuloma
	FACE
	Fibroblastic rheumatism
	Foreign body granuloma
	Granuloma annulare
	Nephrogenic systemic fibrosis
	Phalangeal pads[a]
	Rheumatoid nodule and palisading granuloma
	Sarcoidosis
Miscellaneous	Accessory tragus, supernumerary nipple
	Dupuytren's disease
	Fox-Fordyce disease
	Palmar papules (basaloid follicular hamartoma, Darier's disease, Cowden disease, oxalate deposits, etc.)
	Pearly penile papules

FACE facial Afro-Caribbean childhood eruption
[a]The surface is usually altered

D. Lipsker, *Clinical Examination and Differential Diagnosis of Skin Lesions*,
DOI 10.1007/978-2-8178-0411-8_31, © Springer-Verlag France 2013

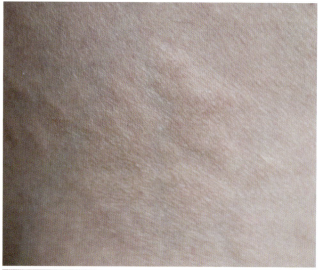

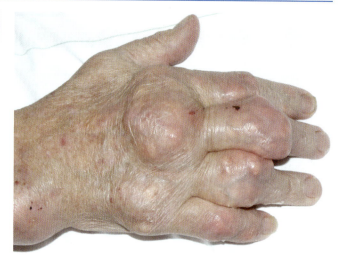

Fig. 31.3 Flesh-colored nodule with whitish-yellow areas. Gouty tophus

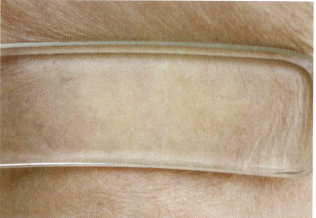

Fig. 31.1 Flesh-colored plaque, slightly erythematous. Nephrogenic systemic fibrosis. Note the yellow coloration on diascopy

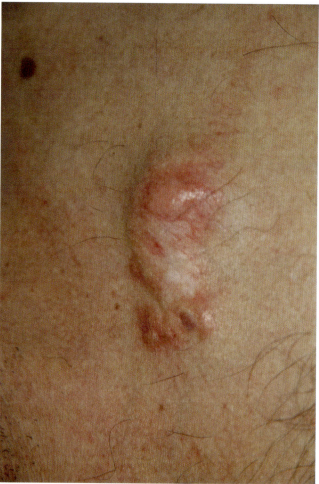

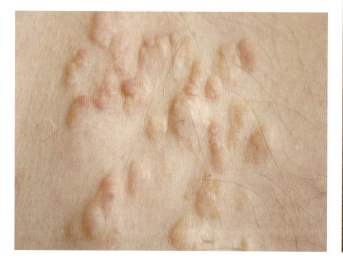

Fig. 31.2 Grouped papules and plaques involving the thigh. Nevus lipomatosus. These lesions are very soft on palpation. Their coloration is characteristic: between normal skin color and *yellow*

Fig. 31.4 Multilobulated telangiectatic nodule with different shades of color. Dermatofibrosarcoma. The multilobulated appearance is very common in the course of this slow-growing tumor

Do Not Miss

Single lesion: benign or malignant skin tumors and metastases.

Multiple lesions: consider an overload disease or a granulomatous disease. In this particular situation, especially when lesions are located on the face, clinicians should suspect and be able to diagnose syndromes such as Cowden, Muir Torre, Gardner's, and Birt-Hogg-Dubé. Those syndromes confer a predisposition to develop visceral cancers.

Common

Nevus, skin tag, and fibroma.

Keratotic papules should be considered separately from other papules. Certain very common disorders are keratotic and should be recognized, i.e., keratosis pilaris, warts, corns, seborrheic keratosis, and also squamous cell carcinoma and actinic keratoses.

Table 31.2 Main causes of palpable solid lesions of the same color as normal skin, with alteration of the skin surface

Genodermatoses	Cowden disease
	Darier's disease
	Epidermodysplasia verruciformis
Non-melanocytic nevus and tumors	Angiokeratoma (usually violaceous)
	Benign and malignant, epithelial and adnexal tumors: carcinomas, hidradenoma papilliferum, actinic keratosis, seborrheic keratosis, porokeratoses, syringocystadenoma, etc.
	Cutaneous horn
	Dermatofibrosarcoma
	Digital fibrokeratoma
	Kerinokeratosis papulosa
	Knuckle pads (pachydermodactyly)
	Nevus comedonicus
	Nevus sebaceous
	Verrucous epidermal nevus
Infections	Crusted scabies
	Warts (common, mosaic, etc.)
Miscellaneous	Acral keratoses (acrokeratosis verruciformis of Hopf and Darier's disease, stucco keratosis, hyperkeratosis lenticularis perstans (also known as "Flegel's disease"), keratoelastoidosis marginalis, Cowden disease)
	Filiform hyperkeratosis and myelomatous spicules
	Ichthyosis
	Keratodermas
	Keratosis pilaris
	Lymphedema papules in mossy foot disease
	Open comedo and dilated pore of Winer
	Perforating dermatoses (Kyrle's disease, perforating collagenoma, perforating folliculitis, perforating serpiginous elastosis, pseudo-PXE related to D-penicillamine, etc.)

PXE pseudoxanthoma elasticum

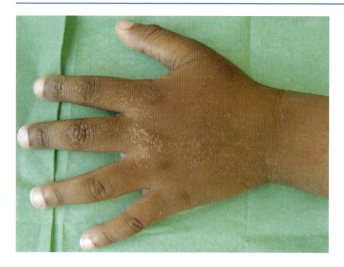

Fig. 31.5 Multiple submillimeter-sized papules. Lichen nitidus. If in doubt, a histopathological evaluation would reveal a typical picture

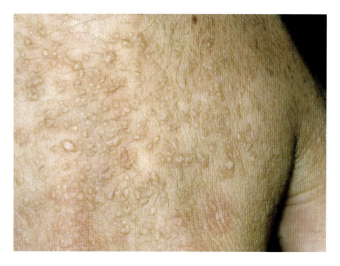

Fig. 31.6 Multiple keratotic papules on the back of the hands. Darier's disease

Do Not Miss

Single lesions: benign and malignant skin tumors.

Multiple lesions: in this particular situation, especially when lesions are located on the face, clinicians should suspect and be able to diagnose syndromes such as Cowden, Muir Torre, Gardner's, and Birt-Hogg-Dubé, which are associated with increased risk of visceral cancers, just as myelomatous spicules point to the possibility of associated myeloma. Mechanical hands in dermatopolymyositis are keratotic, just as acrokeratosis paraneoplastica (Bazex syndrome), which usually reveals an ENT cancer.

Common

Cutaneous horns, keratosis pilaris, seborrheic keratosis, and actinic keratosis.

Brown, Black, Blue, or Gray Palpable Lesions

32

These lesions are usually isolated and rarely multiple. Although precisely identifying the primary lesion is essential in establishing a differential diagnosis, it is important to note that there is significant overlapping between a papule, a plaque, and a nodule. Indeed, a single disorder can manifest simultaneously or successively as each of these lesions, either through their growth or confluence, or by nature. Since it is vital to diagnose melanoma and other pigmented cancers, a biopsy is indicated in case of the slightest doubt. This situation also requires that clinical examination sometimes be completed by a careful inspection using a magnifier lens or a dermatoscope. The latter may provide additional elements that can help avoid biopsy in some instances. However, histopathological examination remains the "gold standard" for establishing the precise diagnosis of any skin tumor. Certain lesions may have a purple coloration and thus reflect a dermal inflammation (e.g., lichen planus) or an angiomatous proliferation (e.g., Kaposi's disease). Certain violaceous palpable lesions are angiokeratomas. When they are numerous and distributed over the "underwear" area, they can reflect an overload disease such as Fabry disease, which, if diagnosed early, can be treated by enzyme replacement therapy. Serious renal, cardiac, and/or cerebral complications can thus be avoided.

Botryomycoma
Bowenoid papulosis
Cutaneous B-cell lymphoma
Dermatofibrosarcoma
Dermatosis papulosis nigra (Castellani's disease)
Glomus tumor (and glomangiomatosis)
Hemangioma (cavernous and verrucous)
Hidrocystoma
Kaposi's disease
Leukemias (particularly acute myeloid leukemia 4 and 5, NK-lymphoma, and dendritic plasmacytoid CD56-positive lymphomas)
Melanocytic tumors (melanoma, nevus, etc.)
Metastases (particularly of melanoma)
Open comedo and dilated pore of Winer
Pigmented viral wart
Purple papules in lichen planus, granuloma annulare, and collagen vascular diseases
Seborrheic keratosis
Skin cancers and precancerous lesions (pigmented basal cell carcinoma, pigmented Bowen's disease, pigmented actinic keratosis, pigmented eccrine porocarcinoma, etc.)
Urticaria pigmentosa

Box 32.1 Main Causes of Brown, Black, Blue, or Gray Palpable Lesions

Acanthosis nigricans
Acroangiodermatitis (pseudo-Kaposi's sarcoma, arteriovenous fistula)
Acrochordon or skin tag
Angiokeratoma (usually violaceous)
Angiolymphoid hyperplasia with eosinophilia and Kimura disease
Angiosarcoma
Black piedra
Blue nevus

Do Not Miss

Isolated lesions: melanoma and other pigmented cancers.

Multiple lesions (rare): metastases, namely, of melanoma, and leukemia cutis, as well as urticaria pigmentosa in cutaneous and systemic mastocytoses (usually macular), can have a brown coloration.

Common

Nevus, fibroma, and acrochordon.

D. Lipsker, *Clinical Examination and Differential Diagnosis of Skin Lesions*,
DOI 10.1007/978-2-8178-0411-8_32, © Springer-Verlag France 2013

Mechanisms underlying the white color of these lesions have been addressed in Chap. 3, dedicated to macules. The most common white palpable lesions are cysts, molluscum contagiosum, and sebaceous hyperplasias. Other lesions are the manifestations of metabolic disorders such as gouty tophus or calcinoses; the latter may occur, for example, in patients with connective tissue diseases.

Box 33.1 Main Causes of White, Solid, Palpable Lesions

Achromic melanoma

Acne

Cutaneous calcinosis

Dysplastic nevus (rare)

Keratosis pilaris

Lichen nitidus

Milia seeds and other epidermoid cysts

Molluscum contagiosum

Nits (hair)

Papular elastorrhexis

Sebaceous hyperplasia (yellow-white)

Tophus

White lentiginosis

White papulosis (or clear cell/pagetoid papulosis)

White piedra (hair)

Do Not Miss

An achromic melanoma should not be ignored.

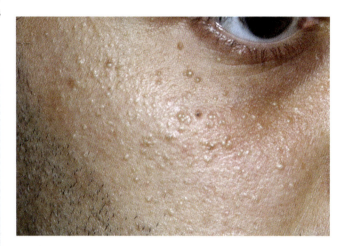

Fig. 33.1 White papules. Milia seeds. These are one type of microcysts

D. Lipsker, *Clinical Examination and Differential Diagnosis of Skin Lesions*,
DOI 10.1007/978-2-8178-0411-8_33, © Springer-Verlag France 2013

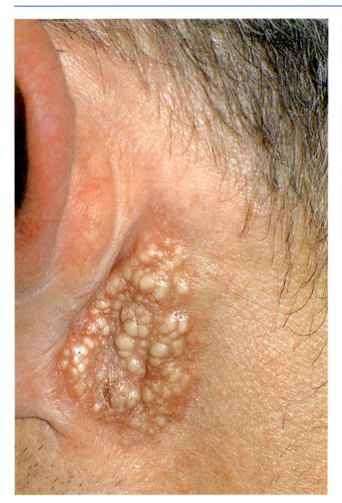

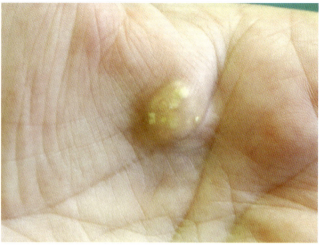

Fig. 33.3 Yellow nodule with white spots. Cutaneous calcinosis in systemic sclerosis

Fig. 33.2 Multilobulated white plaque, consisting of multiple hemispherical papules. Colloid milium. The location behind the ear is characteristic

Mechanisms underlying the yellow color of these lesions have been addressed in Chap. 3, dedicated to macules. Upon initial clinical evaluation, yellow circumscribed lesions can immediately be differentiated from a more diffuse yellow dyschromia (such as carotenoid pigmentation, certain drug intoxications or, rarely, diffuse plane xanthomatosis). In the case of yellow circumscribed lesions, keratoses are easily identified by the rough nature of the primary lesion. Although purpura evolves through a transient yellow coloration, it is easily diagnosed through history taking and the presence of associated lesions. When diagnosing other yellow infiltrated lesions, skin biopsy is usually mandatory, as well as special coloration techniques such as orcein staining, which allows visualization of elastic fibers and thioflavin T for identification of amyloid deposits. Immunohistochemistry techniques are also required for characterizing either a lymphomatous or histiocytic infiltrate. Certain yellow palpable lesions are the morphological expression of pseudoxanthoma elasticum. This rare disorder of the elastic tissue may explain an early atheromatosis and thus explain so far unresolved episodes of coronaropathy and strokes in a young patient. In neonates, the most common causes of a yellow papule or plaque are sebaceous hamartoma, juvenile xanthogranuloma, and mastocytoma.

Box 34.1 Main Causes of Yellow, Solid, Palpable Lesions

Amyloidosis (nodular, usually orange-yellow)

Colloid milium

Cysts (usually white or skin-colored)

Farber lipogranulomatosis

Histiocytic lesions: Langerhans cell histiocytosis, normo-lipemic xanthoma (Erdheim-Chester disease, normolipemic planar xanthoma, necrobiotic xanthogranuloma, diffuse plane xanthomatosis, etc.)

Infections: tertiary syphilis, lupus vulgaris

Juvenile xanthogranuloma

Kerinokeratosis papulosa

Lipid metaplasia

Lipoid proteinosis (hyalinosis cutis et mucosae or Urbach-Wiethe disease)

Lymphomas, leukemias

Mastocytoma

Necrobiosis lipoidica

Pseudoxanthoma elasticum

Sarcoidosis

Sebaceous hyperplasia (yellow-white)

Sebaceous nevus

Tophus

Xanthelasma

Xanthomas (eruptive, tendinous, tuberous)

D. Lipsker, *Clinical Examination and Differential Diagnosis of Skin Lesions*,
DOI 10.1007/978-2-8178-0411-8_34, © Springer-Verlag France 2013

Do Not Miss

Granulomatous disorders should not be ignored, whether infectious (i.e., mycobacterial infections, tertiary (or late) syphilis) or not (e.g., sarcoidosis), as well as cellular infiltrates in histiocytoses or, rarely, in certain lymphomas and leukemias. The diagnosis of eruptive xanthomas in patients with hyperlipidemia, whether affected or not by Zieve's syndrome, can be a life-threatening emergency.

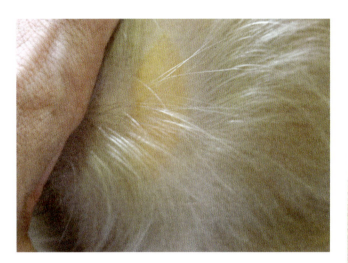

Fig. 34.1 Barely raised yellow plaque, located on the scalp. Nevus sebaceous

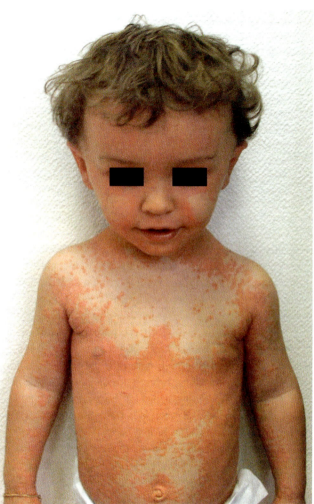

Fig. 34.3 Confluent, orange papules, and plaques. Pityriasis rubra pilaris. Note the intervals of unaffected skin on the cheeks and trunk, very typical of this rare disorder

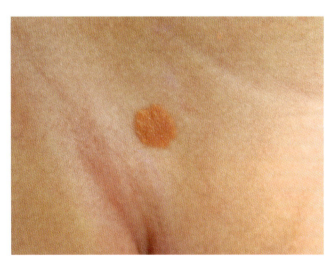

Fig. 34.2 Orange papule. Juvenile xanthogranuloma

Non-purpuric, palpable red lesions are very common and have a great number of causes. They are often the consequence of cutaneous inflammatory diseases. Thus dermatological and extracutaneous associated signs, as well as context, are an important part of differential diagnosis. The "relevant" contexts are numerous and varied: neutropenia and immune deficiency, newly taken drugs, and cold triggering, to name a few. Among possible causes are severe infections (such as septicemias) and cutaneous manifestations in leukemias: the clinical situation of these patients must therefore be carefully analyzed. Indeed, these lesions can easily be trivialized, being very common with very familiar causes, such as insect bites or urticaria.

Certain papular inflammatory dermatoses can be clinically identified, for example, typical lichen papules. In such a case, they have a characteristic purple coloration and are flat, polygonal, and covered with fine white striations, called "Wickham's striae." They are pruritic. In case of lesions of secondary syphilis, a perilesional collarette surrounding the papule is very suggestive of this diagnosis, especially when lesions are located on extremities.

Neutrophilic dermatoses (i.e., Sweet syndrome), vasculitides, and erythema multiforme are possible causes of multiple, eruptive, edematous plaques.

Inflammatory lesions located in the hypodermis (deep-seated nodules, or "nouures" in French terminology) reflect an affection either of the adipose lobules (lobular panniculitis), of the inter-adipose septa (septal panniculitis), or of hypodermal vessels (either veins or arteries).

Papules often have an altered surface and produce intricate lesions which are discussed later on, i.e., papulopustules, scaly papules, and necrotic papules.

Box 35.1 Main Causes of Erythematous Papules

Acne
Atypical fibroxanthoma
Botryomycoma
Burn caused by marine animals and plants
Chilblain
Cutaneous Kikuchi disease
Cutaneous manifestations in septicemias
Eosinophilic folliculitis (usually pustular)
EPPER (eosinophilic, polymorphic, and pruritic eruption associated with radiotherapy)
Eruptive xanthoma (pink)
Erythema elevatum diutinum (on the back of the hands)
Fibroblastic rheumatism
Flea bites
Folliculitis caused by infection with *Malassezia* (usually pustular)
Foreign body granuloma
Gianotti-Crosti syndrome
Gluteal granuloma
Gottron's papules in dermatomyositis (back of the hands)
Granuloma annulare (which generally merges into annular lesions)
Grover's disease (often papulovesicular)
Hordeolum (or sty) and chalazion
Insect bite and sting
Kaposi's disease
Lymphomatoid papulosis
Multicentric reticulohistiocytosis (back of the hands)
Perforating elastoma (that merge into arciform lesions)
Pityriasis lichenoides
Prurigo
Rickettsioses
Rosacea
Ruby spots (or cherry angioma)
Sarcoidosis (often annular)
Scabies
Secondary syphilis
Urticaria

D. Lipsker, *Clinical Examination and Differential Diagnosis of Skin Lesions*,
DOI 10.1007/978-2-8178-0411-8_35, © Springer-Verlag France 2013

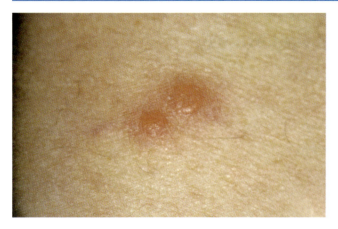

Fig. 35.1 Succulent (i.e., "impregnated with fluid") erythematous papules on an erythematous macule. Prurigo

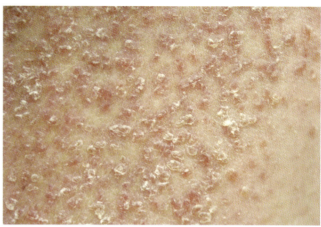

Fig. 35.4 Scaly and keratotic red papules. Keratosis lichenoides chronica. Note the reticulated and linear arrangement of the lesions

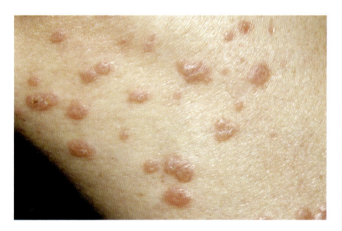

Fig. 35.2 Red papules. Lichen (planus)

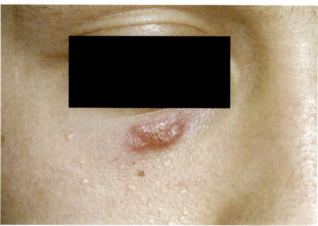

Fig. 35.5 Red papule with a scaly and keratotic center. Leishmaniasis. Also note the surrounding white hemispherical papules, i.e., milia seeds, as well as the two small nevi

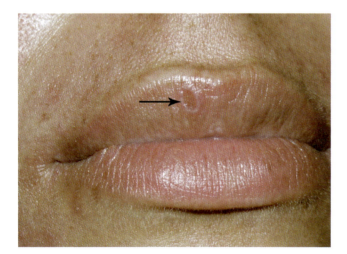

Fig. 35.3 Annular papule with central erosion, located on the vermilion border of the upper lip (*arrow*). Lichen

Box 35.2 Main Causes of Erythematous Plaques and Nodules

Acne (conglobata, pyoderma faciale)

Adult onset Still's disease

Angioendotheliomatoses

Angiolymphoid hyperplasia with eosinophilia

Arboviruses

Chilblain

Cylindromas

Erysipela and cellulitis

Erythema elevatum diutinum

Erythema multiforme

Erythema nodosum

Furuncle, anthrax

Furunculoid myiasis

Granuloma annulare (deep-seated)

Granuloma faciale (Lever type)

Hemangioma

Hidradenitis suppurativa, dissecting cellulitis

Infectious cellulitis

Inflammatory epidermoid cyst

Insect bite and sting

Jessner-Kanof disease (located on the face, often annular, a dermal variant of lupus erythematosus)

Kaposi's disease

Lupus erythematosus

Lymphomas and leukemias

Mycobacterial infection (particularly *M. marinum*)

NERDS nodules (nodules, eosinophilia, rheumatism, dermatitis, swelling)

Nodular vasculitis (erythema induratum of Bazin)

Orf and milker's nodule

Panniculitis (all types)

Polymorphous light eruption (face)

Pruritic urticarial papules and plaques of pregnancy

Pseudolymphoma

Relapsing polychondritis (cartilaginous areas)

Rheumatoid nodules

Sarcoma, angiosarcoma

Sporotrichosis

Sweet syndrome and other neutrophilic dermatoses

Urticaria

Vasculitides (medium to large vessels, as well as granulomatous forms), hypocomplementemic vasculitis, and acute hemorrhagic edema of infancy

Wells syndrome (eosinophilic cellulitis)

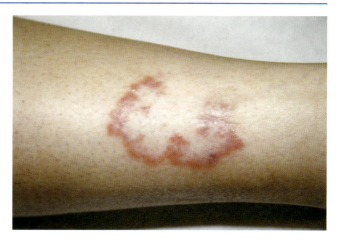

Fig. 35.6 Arciform erythematous plaque. Leprosy

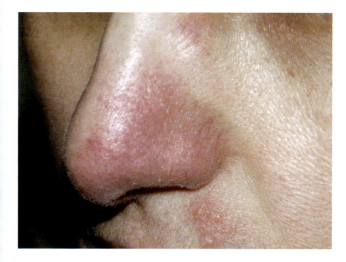

Fig. 35.7 Angiomatous and telangiectatic plaque. Sarcoidosis

Do Not Miss

Bacterial and fungal septicemias and severe viral infections (arboviruses). Cutaneous manifestation of many systemic diseases: vasculitides, neutrophilic diseases, connective tissue diseases, and histiocytoses.

Common

Insect bite and sting, folliculitis, acne, rosacea.

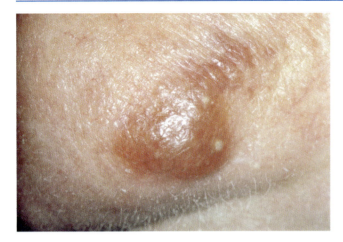

Fig. 35.8 Reddish-brown nodule. Nodular amyloidosis. The evolution towards anetoderma is characteristic. This disorder belongs to the same disease spectrum as cutaneous plasmocytoma; it is associated with systemic amyloidosis in approximately 15 % of cases

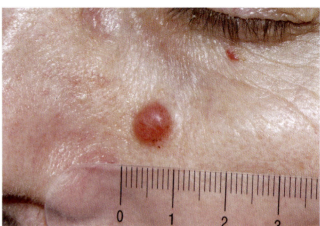

Fig. 35.11 Erythematous nodule. Merkel cell carcinoma (also known as neuroendocrine carcinoma of the skin)

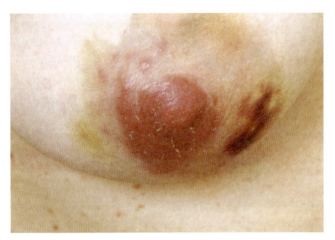

Fig. 35.9 Erythematous plaque involving the areola. Lymphocytoma induced by infection with *Borrelia*. Note the perilesional ecchymosis following fine-needle aspiration biopsy; the lesion being indurated and frequently located in the nipple-areolar area, these patients are sometimes referred to breast care and undergo fine-needle aspiration biopsy

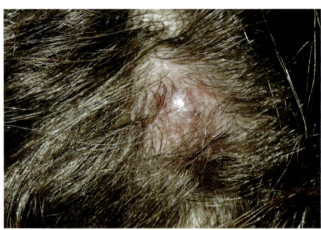

Fig. 35.12 Telangiectatic nodule of the scalp causing hair loss. Metastasis of kidney cancer

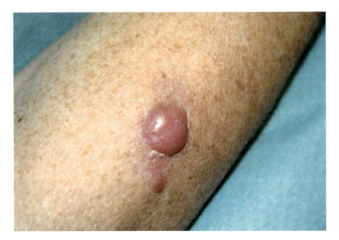

Fig. 35.10 Erythematous nodule without alteration of the cutaneous surface. Cutaneous, marginal zone, B-cell lymphoma

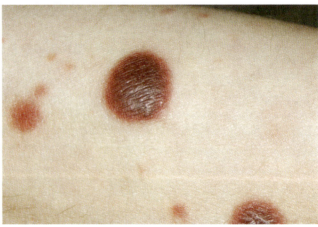

Fig. 35.13 Macules, papules, and red plaques without alteration of the skin surface. Leukemia

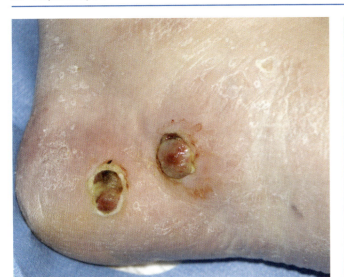

Fig. 35.14 Ulcerated nodules. Kaposi's disease. These types of lesions cannot be clearly identified from a clinical point of view; many diagnostic hypotheses can be discussed and biopsy is essential

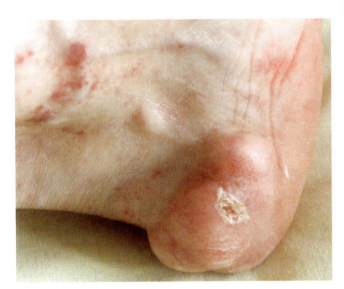

Fig. 35.15 Multilobulated nodule of the heel. Rheumatoid nodule. Also note an isolated rheumatoid nodule, immediately above

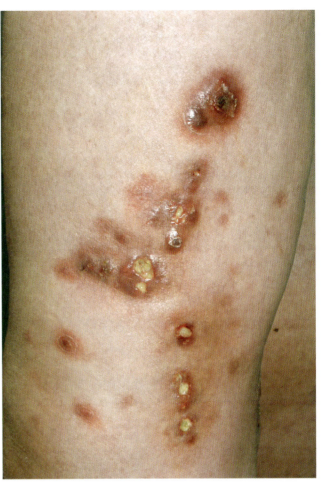

Fig. 35.16 Fistulated nodules. Infection with *Mycobacterium chelonae* in an immunosuppressed patient. Note the linear arrangement along the lymphatic channels (this type of dissemination is also called sporotrichoid)

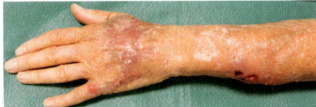

Fig. 35.17 Erythematous plaques and nodules with purulent fistulas, gummy ulcers, and crusts. Infection with *Scytalidium* in an immunosuppressed patient (having received a transplant and taking immunosuppressants). Also note the dermatoporosis

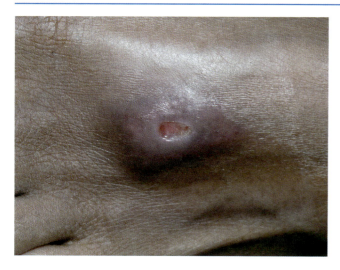

Fig. 35.18 Ulcerated nodule. BCGitis

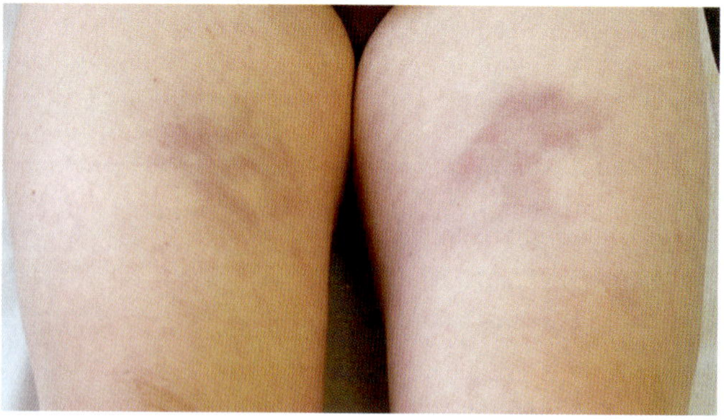

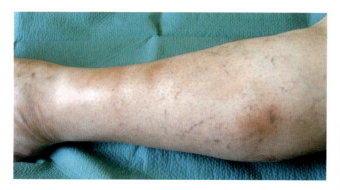

Fig. 35.19 Erythematous and pigmented infiltrated plaques on the leg. Lipomembranous fat necrosis associated with lipodermatosclerosis. Note the signs of venous insufficiency that are almost always associated: phlebectases and varicosities

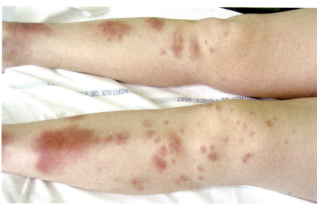

Fig. 35.20 Violaceous infiltrated plaques of the anterior-internal part of the thighs. Panniculitis caused by cold temperature (cold panniculitis)

Fig. 35.21 Papules, plaques, and erythematous deep-seated nodules. Sweet syndrome in a patient with Crohn's disease. "Deep-seated" Sweet syndrome of the lower limbs cannot be distinguished from erythema nodosa (cf. Figs. 4.21 and 4.22)

Follicular Papules and Keratosis Pilaris

36

Table 36.1 Main causes of follicular papules and keratosis pilaris

Infections	Acne
	Folliculitis and pseudofolliculitis
	Follicular syphilids
	Follicular tuberculids
	Rash of measles
Immune-related	Dermatomyositis with follicular hyperkeratosis (Wong's dermatomyositis)
	Follicular eruption of atopic dermatitis
	Follicular variants of acute generalized exanthematous pustuloses (usually pustular)
Dermatoses and general diseases	Darier's disease
	Follicular lichen planus
	Follicular mucinosis
	Follicular psoriasis (particularly in children)
	Folliculocentric Langerhans cell histiocytosis
	Grover's disease
	Kyrle's disease
	Lichen nitidus
	Pilotropic mycosis fungoides
	Pityriasis rubra pilaris
Metabolic causes	Chronic kidney disease
	Disorders of vitamin A metabolism (phrynoderma secondary to vitamin A deficiency)
	Keratosis pilaris due to nutritional deficiency
External factors	Follicular contact dermatitis
	Oils

Table 36.1 (continued)

Hereditary or congenital causes	Follicular hyperkeratosis associated with congenital keratoderma in ichthyosis vulgaris (AD)
	Jadassohn-Lewandowsky syndrome (pachyonychia congenita)
	Marie Unna's hereditary hypotrichosis (hereditary trichodysplasia)
	Monilethrix
	Pilar (hair) aplasia (atrichia congenita with cysts)
	Pili torti
	Scarring keratosis pilaris:
	Keratosis pilaris decalvans (Siemens syndrome)
	KID
	IFAP syndrome
	Hereditary mucoepithelial dysplasia
	Ulerythema ophryogenes and Brocq's keratosis pilaris rubra atrophicans faciei (sometimes as part of Noonan's or Fairbank's or cardiofaciocutaneous syndromes)
	Vermiculate atrophoderma of the cheeks (can be one of the signs of Nicolau-Balus syndrome or Rombo syndrome)
Simple keratosis pilaris	Cutis anserina ("goose flesh")
	Essential
	In patients with atopy
	Miscellaneous

AD autosomal dominant, *KID* keratitis, ichthyosis, deafness, *IFAP* ichthyosis follicularis, alopecia, photophobia

D. Lipsker, *Clinical Examination and Differential Diagnosis of Skin Lesions*,
DOI 10.1007/978-2-8178-0411-8_36, © Springer-Verlag France 2013

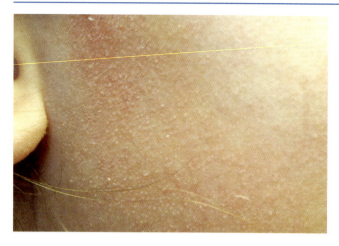

Fig. 36.1 Flesh-colored millimeter-wide papules. Keratosis pilaris. Note the equidistant follicular distribution

Palpable Lesions with a Specific Topography

37.1 Palpable Lesions Located on Extremities

Table 37.1 Main causes of palpable lesions of the extremities

Papules or plaques (normal cutaneous surface)	Keratosis
Acral papular mucinosis	Acrokeratoelastoidosis
APACHE syndrome	Acrokeratosis
Chilblains	Acrokeratosis paraneoplastica (Bazex syndrome)
Erythema elevatum diutinum	Acrokeratosis verruciformis of Hopf in Cowden disease
Erythema multiforme	Darier's disease
Fibroblastic rheumatism	Focal acral hyperkeratosis
Gottron's papules in dermatomyositis	Hyperkeratosis lenticularis perstans (also known as "Flegel's disease")
Granuloma annulare	Keratosis lichenoides chronica
Hereditary progressive mucinous histiocytosis	Kyrle's disease
Mercury poisoning (mainly papulovesicles)	
Multicentric reticulohistiocytosis	Lutz-Lewandowsky disease (epidermodysplasia verruciformis)
Multinucleate cell angiohistiocytoma	Perforating collagenoma
Papular elastolytic giant cell granuloma	Perforating serpiginous elastosis
Self-healing juvenile cutaneous mucinosis	Seborrheic keratosis
	Skin cancers (including actinic keratosis and keratoacanthoma)
	Solitary lichenoid keratosis
	Stucco keratosis
	Superficial actinic porokeratosis
	Warts

APACHE acral pseudolymphomatous angiokeratoma of children

37.2 Periarticular Palpable Lesions

Box 37.1 Main Causes of Periarticular Palpable Lesions

Buschke-Ollendorff syndrome
Chilblains
Chronic bursitis
Cutaneous calcinosis
(Distal) interphalangeal arthritis (Heberden's nodes)
Ehlers-Danlos syndrome
Erythema elevatum diutinum
Erythema multiforme
Exostoses
Fibroblastic rheumatism
Fibrous nodules of acrodermatitis chronica atrophicans
Glomus tumor
Gottron's papules in dermatomyositis
Gout
Granuloma annulare
Hereditary camptodactyly
Intravascular histiocytosis
Juvenile fibromatoses
Knuckle pads
Mafucci-Kast syndrome
Multicentric reticulohistiocytosis
Multinucleate cell angiohistiocytoma
Necrobiosis lipoidica
NERDS syndrome (Nodules, Eosinophilia, Rheumatism, Dermatitis, Swelling)
Nodular fibromatosis
Nodules appearing in endemic treponematoses: pian, bejel
(Para)synovial cysts
Piezogenic papules
Proximal interphalangeal joint arthritis (Bouchard's nodes)
Rheumatoid nodules
Self-healing juvenile cutaneous mucinosis
Synovialomas
Tendinitis, peritendinitis, and chronic tenosynovitis
Xanthomas

D. Lipsker, *Clinical Examination and Differential Diagnosis of Skin Lesions*,
DOI 10.1007/978-2-8178-0411-8_37, © Springer-Verlag France 2013

37.3   Palpable Lesions of the Face and Eyelids

Table 37.2 Main causes of multiple skin-colored or pigmented papules of the face and eyelids

Face	Eyelids
Infections:	*Metabolic causes:*
Lepromatous leprosy	Lipoid proteinosis (hyalinosis cutis et mucosae or Urbach-Wiethe disease)
Molluscum contagiosum	Primary systemic amyloidosis (or Lubarsch-Pick syndrome)
Multiple flat warts	Xanthomatosis of Montgomery
Pseudo-lepromatous leishmaniasis	Xanthelasma
Tumors:	*Infections:*
Actinic keratoses and skin cancers	Flat warts
Angiofibroma and fibrous papule (tuberous sclerosis)	Molluscum contagiosum
Basal cell hamartoma (Gorlin's syndrome)	*Tumors:*
Cylindroma	Hidrocystoma
Facial papules associated with B cell blood disorders	Milium
Hidrocystoma	Skin tags
Keratoacanthoma	Syringomas
Neurofibroma (neurofibromatosis)	Trichilemmoma (Cowden syndrome)
Nevus	
Seborrheic keratoses	
Skin tag (or acrochordon)	
Trichilemmoma (Cowden syndrome)	
Trichodiscoma, fibrofolliculoma, perifollicular fibroma (Birt-Hogg-Dubé syndrome)	
Trichoepithelioma	
Inflammations:	
Acne (microcyst)	
Actinic prurigo	
Micronodular and macronodular sarcoidosis	
Polymorphous light eruption	
Rosacea (particularly granulomatous variants)	
Scleromyxedema	

Palmoplantar keratodermas are a common clinical finding and thus addressed in this chapter. Keratoderma is a scaly and/or keratotic thickening of the palms and/or soles. Keratoderma may affect exclusively the palms, or the soles, or both. The diagnosis of the underlying causative disorder can be difficult, as differential diagnosis includes many different diseases. The acquired forms are more common and may reveal a serious disease such as cancer or lymphoma. They may also be triggered by an infection such as reactive arthritis (i.e., keratoderma blennorrhagica). Frequent causes of keratodermas are dermatophytosis, orthoergic dermatitis, or psoriasis. However, they have many potential causes and they can be one of the signs or early in the course the only sign of a general disease, such as dermatomyositis or hypothyroidism. They also correspond to the acral manifestation of many dermatoses, such as ichthyoses.

Keratoderma can be localized or diffuse. When diffuse, they affect the entire palm and sole. The localized forms can be focal, striated, or punctate. Hence they produce round, keratotic areas of a few millimeters wide. These keratotic areas are described as focal when measuring more than 5–10 mm and punctate when millimeter wide.

They are described as striated when producing linear or reticulated areas and transgredient ("keratoderma transgrediens"), when extending over the palmar and/or plantar area and when the keratosis thus spreads towards the lateral or dorsal parts of hands or feet.

The diagnosis of the numerous variants of congenital keratodermas is based on heredity (AD, AR, or X-linked, mitochondrial, etc.), semiology (diffuse or localized, focal, striated, or punctate), and associated signs (isolated or syndromic). The association of early keratoderma with wooly hair is often the first expression of a hereditary disease of desmosomes, which exposes to a potentially lethal cardiac risk (arrhythmogenic right ventricular cardiomyopathy, left ventricular dilated cardiomyopathy) in patients with Naxos or Carvajal syndromes.

Box 38.1 Main Causes of Acquired Keratodermas and Keratodermas Occurring in Well-Defined Diseases

Mecanogenic causes

Infectious causes

    Crusted scabies

    Mycoses (dermatophytosis)

    Pitted keratolysis caused by *Corynebacterium minutissimum*

    Reactive arthritis

    Secondary syphilis and endemic treponematosis (pian)

    Verrucous tuberculosis

    Warts

Drug-related causes (gold salts, hydantoin, mepacrine, proguanil, mexiletine, alpha-methyldopa, practolol, hydroxyurea, retinoids, streptomycin)

Arsenicals

Hormones

    Climacteric keratoderma (Haxthausen's syndrome)

    Hypothyroidism

    Miscellaneous: pheochromocytoma, pituitary insufficiency, and diabetes

Circulatory causes (lymphedema: elephantiasis verrucosa nostra)

Paraneoplastic causes

    Acrokeratosis paraneoplastica (Bazex syndrome)

    Howel-Evans syndrome

    Tripe palms and acanthosis nigricans

Zinc deficiency

Idiopathic punctate keratosis

Idiopathic punctate keratosis of the folds of the palm

Palmoplantar keratodermas in the context of other dermatoses and diseases (including genodermatoses)

    Cardiofaciocutaneous syndrome

    Christ-Siemens-Touraine syndrome

    Clouston's hidrotic ectodermal dysplasia

    Contact and atopic dermatitis

    Cowden syndrome

    Cutaneous T-cell lymphoma (mycosis fungoides)

(continued)

D. Lipsker, *Clinical Examination and Differential Diagnosis of Skin Lesions*,
DOI 10.1007/978-2-8178-0411-8_38, © Springer-Verlag France 2013

Box 38.1 (continued)

Darier's disease and acrokeratosis verruciformis of Hopf
Dyskeratosis congenita (Zinsser-Cole-Engman syndrome)
Epidermodysplasia verruciformis (of Lutz-Lewandowsky)
Epidermolysis bullosa simplex
Erythrodermas
Gorlin's syndrome
Ichthyoses and bullous congenital ichthyosiform erythro-
derma, erythrokeratodermas
Juvenile palmar dermatitis acquired at swimming pools
Juvenile plantar dermatosis
KID syndrome: keratitis, ichthyosis, and deafness
Kindler syndrome
Lichen planus and lichen nitidus
Mechanic hands in dermatomyositis and keratoses caused
by lupus erythematosus
Naegeli-Franceschetti-Jadassohn syndrome
Pityriasis rubra pilaris
Porokeratosis palmaris et plantaris disseminata
Psoriasis
Reticulate and pigmented dermopathy
Weary-Kindler syndrome

Table 38.1 lists the main hereditary keratodermas, but is incomplete and evolutive since molecular genetics have enabled the reclassification of a large number of these diseases. However, it is difficult to propose a simple yet logical classification. Most of these disorders include other signs for which they would be categorized among genetic diseases accompanied by keratoderma (cf. Box 38.1).

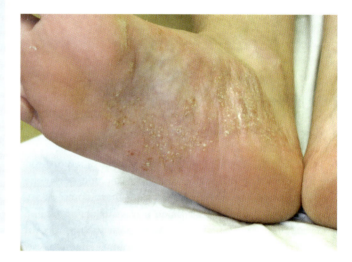

Fig. 38.2 Pustular and scaly mid-plantar keratoderma. Palmoplantar pustulosis. Note the characteristic extension to the lateral part of the foot, as well as the spared forefoot and heel

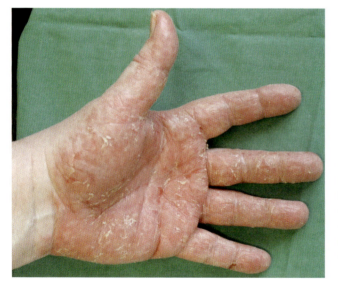

Fig. 38.1 Scaly and erythematous, fissured keratoderma. Psoriasis

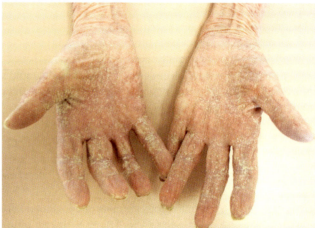

Fig. 38.3 Profuse scaly keratoderma. Scabies. It is essential to look for furrows

Table 38.1 Main hereditary keratodermas

Autosomal dominant keratodermas (AD)

Diffuse	Greither's keratoderma
	Huriez syndrome
	Keratoderma of Camisa
	Keratoderma with tonotubular keratin
	Norrbotten-type keratoderma
	Olmsted syndrome
	Thost-Unna palmoplantar keratoderma
	Vohwinkel keratoderma
	Vörner's keratoderma
Focal and striated	Focal palmoplantar keratoderma
	Hereditary cutaneous horns with bullae
	Hopp's syndrome
	Howel-Evans syndrome
	Pachyonychia congenita type I
	Pachyonychia congenita type II
	Striated keratoderma
Punctate	Acrokeratoelastoidosis (of Mendes da Costa)
	Focal acral hyperkeratosis
	Punctate keratoderma
	Spiny keratoderma (punctate porokeratosis)

Autosomal recessive keratodermas (AR)

Diffuse	Bureau-Barrière-Thomas syndrome
	Epidermolytic keratodermas
	Keratoderma Gamborg-Nielsen's type
	Keratoderma of Méléda's type
	KLICK syndrome
	Naxos disease
	Papillon-Lefèvre syndrome
	Schöpf-Schulz-Passarge syndrome
Focal	Carvajal syndrome
	Richner-Hanhart syndrome (tyrosinemia type II)

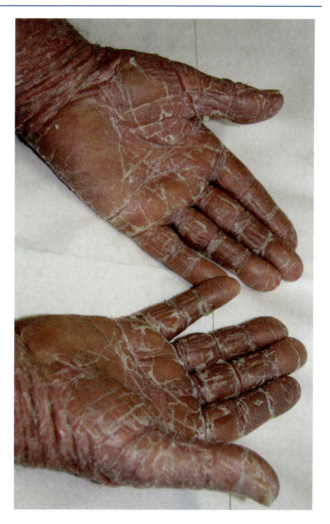

Fig. 38.5 *Orange*-colored keratoderma. Pityriasis rubra pilaris. This *orange-yellow* coloration is characteristic. Also note the fissures

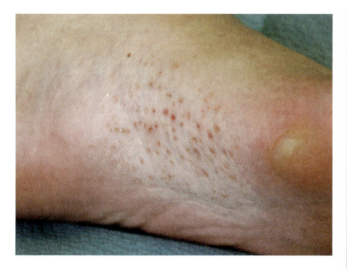

Fig. 38.4 Acquired papular punctate keratoderma. Lichen. Syphilis must always be ruled out in the presence of collarette scaling

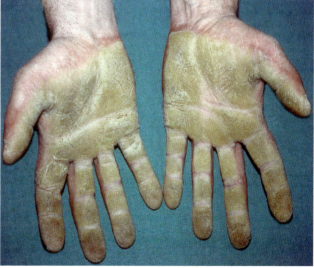

Fig. 38.6 Congenital, homogeneous, thick, *yellow*, diffuse keratoderma. Thost-Unna's disease. Note the peripheral erythematous border

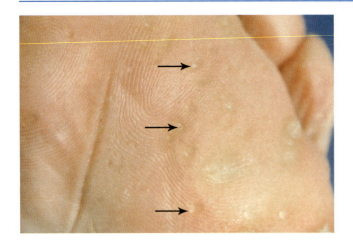

Fig. 38.7 Punctate keratoderma (*arrows*)

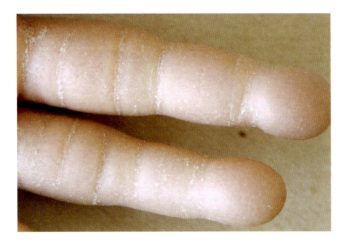

Fig. 38.8 Keratoderma with ainhumoid retraction. Vohwinkel syndrome with ichthyosis. Note the circumferential retraction of the fingers that can sometimes lead to amputations. This denomination is related to the similar appearance described in ainhum

Acquired Keratoderma

May reveal a cancer (acrokeratosis paraneoplastica), a lymphoma, or certain infections such as reactive arthritis, syphilis, or scabies. Other significant causes are arsenicism, hypothyroidism, mechanic hands in dermatomyositis with antisynthetase antibodies, nutritional deficiencies, and Cowden syndrome.

Congenital Keratoderma

Many variants exist, some of which can be present at birth. Focal autosomal recessive keratoderma in patients with Richner-Hanhart syndrome (tyrosinemia type II) should not be overlooked. It can be managed with an appropriate diet, restricted in tyrosine and phenylalanine. Other keratodermas can be associated with visceral or cutaneous cancers or significant diseases such as cardiopathies (Naxos disease, Carvajal disease).

Common

Mechanical causes, dermatophytosis, psoriasis, and dermatitis

Intricate Palpable Lesions

The association between erythematous lesions and scaling/desquamation is very common in many skin disorders (i.e., erythematous macules, papules and/or plaques, associated with scales). The causes of these lesions are quite numerous, as illustrated in Table 39.1. The various types of scaling are described in Chap. 41.

Table 39.1 Main causes of scaly erythematous lesions

Type of lesion		Main causes
Non-excoriated lesions	Predominance of papules	Hailey-Hailey disease
		Impetigo
		Lichen planus
		Langerhans cell histiocytosis
		Lymphomatoid papulosis
		Mammary and extramammary Paget's disease
		Necrolytic migratory erythema: glucagonoma syndrome, acrodermatitis enteropathica, and other deficiency dermatoses
		Nummular dermatitis
		Pityriasis lichenoides
		Pityriasis rosea (of Gibert)
		Psoriasis (guttate)
		Secondary syphilis
		Viral exanthemas (scaling often secondary: measles, rubella, etc.)
	Predominance of plaques	Bazex syndrome (acrokeratosis paraneoplastica)
		Darier's disease
		Dermatophytosis (all sites)
		Skin cancers (superficial basal cell carcinoma, Bowen's disease)
		Dermatomyositis
		Ichthyosis (all types)
		Keratosis lichenoides
		Lichen striatus
		Linear verrucous nevus
		Lupus erythematosus
		Mycosis fungoides (and other variants: Woringer-Kolopp and Ketron-Goodman diseases)
		Paraneoplastic dermatosis characterized by scaly erythematous lesions
		Parapsoriasis (small and large plaque)
		Pellagra
		Photosensitivity and chronic photosensitivity dermatitis syndromes
		Pityriasis rubra pilaris
		Psoriasis
		Reactive arthritis

(continued)

D. Lipsker, *Clinical Examination and Differential Diagnosis of Skin Lesions*, DOI 10.1007/978-2-8178-0411-8_39, © Springer-Verlag France 2013

Table 39.1 (continued)

Type of lesion		Main causes
Excoriated lesions	Multiple excoriations	Atopic dermatitis
		Dermatitis herpetiformis
		Dyshidrotic eczema
		Erythroderma
		HTLV1-associated infective dermatitis
		Lichenification (varying degrees of excoriation)
		Most pruritic dermatoses (pruritus ⇒ scratching ⇒ excoriations)
		Neurodermatitis
		Scabies
		Stasis dermatitis
	Few excoriations	Allergic contact dermatitis
		Darier's disease
		Eczema craquelé
		Hailey-Hailey disease
		Irritant contact dermatitis
		Juvenile palmar dermatitis acquired at swimming pools
		Juvenile plantar dermatosis
		Langerhans cell histiocytosis
		Leiner-Moussous disease
		Perioral dermatitis
		Seborrheic dermatitis
		Lichen striatus
		Linear and verrucous epidermal nevus
		Otitis externa
		Paget's disease
		Photosensitivity and chronic photosensitivity dermatitis syndromes

HTLV Human T-cell lymphoma virus

Do Not Miss

Acrokeratosis paraneoplastica and other syndromes indicative of visceral cancers (e.g., of the pancreas) should be kept in mind. Clinicians should consider mycosis fungoides and follicular mucinosis. Other diseases that can be scaly and erythematous are reactive arthritis, glucagonoma, acrodermatitis enteropathica, and other dermatoses induced by various deficiencies (particularly deficiencies in vitamin B and essential fatty acids), as well as connective tissue diseases (lupus erythematosus, dermatomyositis).

Diseases that should also be kept in mind are syphilis and scabies.

In the presence of a single lesion, consider Bowen's disease, basal cell carcinoma, and Paget's disease.

Common

Dermatitis (all types), dermatophytosis, psoriasis, Gibert's pityriasis rosea, scabies, seborrheic dermatitis, stasis dermatitis, and lichenification. Carcinomas in the elderly

Box 39.1 Main Causes of Necrotic Papules

CD8+ epidermotropic cytotoxic T-cell lymphoma (TIA+, perforin+)

Facial papules in patients with B-cell disorders

Inoculation diseases: rickettsioses, tularemia, etc.

Kikuchi disease (cutaneous)

Lymphomatoid papulosis and anaplastic lymphomas

Pityriasis lichenoides

Syphilids

Tuberculids

Vasculitides

γδ Lymphomas

Do Not Miss

Lymphoma, syphilis, tuberculosis, and inoculation diseases

Box 39.2 Main Causes of Papulopustules

Acne

Arthrocutaneous syndrome

Behçet's disease

Drug eruptions

Endocarditis

Folliculitis

Neonatal listeriosis

Pustular vasculitis

Septicemia (due to *Gonococcus/Meningococcus/Staphylococcus*, etc.)

Sweet syndrome and other neutrophilic dermatoses

Box 39.3 Main Causes of Papulovesicles

Autoimmune bullous dermatoses

Dermatitis (all forms)

Grover's disease

Herpes virus (e.g., chickenpox) and certain Coxsackie virus infections

Insect bite and sting

Mercury poisoning (particularly palms)

Pityriasis lichenoides

Prurigo (particularly the acute variant)

Do Not Miss

Septicemia and endocarditis

Do Not Miss

Viral infections (herpes) and autoimmune bullous dermatosis

Common

Acne and folliculitis

Common

Dermatitis

Cutaneous Sclerosis

Skin is described as sclerotic when it has lost its suppleness and can no longer be folded. Sclerosis is usually associated with atrophy ("scleroatrophy"), as observed in scars for example. Widespread sclerosis is disabling. Depending on its location, it can lead to significant reduction in respiratory or articular amplitudes, thus causing definite functional impairment. The mouth opening can be reduced and sexual activity may be impossible. Secondary and lesional localized sclerosis, such as in certain carcinomas (e.g., morpheiform basal cell carcinoma), must be distinguished from primarily sclerosing disorders such as systemic sclerosis. One of the first signs of acrosclerosis in a patient with systemic sclerosis is the decline and subsequent disappearance of palmar creases on the dorsa of the second phalange. Cutaneous sclerosis can be the manifestation of intoxication. Hence, exposure to toxic substances must always be looked for through history taking (silica, cocaine, etc.). Neonatal scleroses are caused by rare disorders that are listed in Table 40.1.

POEMS (polyneuropathy, organomegaly, endocrinopathy, monoclonal component, skin lesion)

Postinjection scleroderma-like panniculitis (due to injections of vitamin K1, B12, and progestagens)

Scirrhous carcinoma

Scleredema of Buschke

Sclerema neonatorum

Scleroatrophic syndrome of Huriez

Scleroderma-like congenital atrophies (Werner syndrome, acrogeria, acrosclerotic poikilodermas) (cf. Table 40.1)

Sclerodermiform leukemic infiltration

Scleromyxedema

Sclerotic amyloid infiltration

Sclerotic variants of acrodermatitis chronica atrophicans

Sharp syndrome

Spanish toxic oil syndrome

Stasis dermatitis

Systemic sclerosis

Box 40.1 Main Causes of Sclerosis

Atrophoderma (of Pierini and Pasini)

Carcinoid syndrome

Chronic radiodermatitis

Cocainomania

Eosinophilia-myalgia syndrome (L-tryptophane)

Eosinophilic fasciitis (Shulman's syndrome)

Fibroblastic rheumatism (sclerodactyly)

Graft-versus-host reaction (GVRH), sclerodermiform variant

H syndrome

Lichen sclerosus

Metabolic causes (phenylketonuria, glycogenoses, porphyria cutanea tarda, diabetes [Rozenbloom sign], scleredema diutinum)

Morphea

Morpheiform basal cell carcinoma

Nephrogenic systemic fibrosis

Pachydermoperiostosis.

Do Not Miss

Sclerosis is a hallmark of systemic sclerosis. Differential diagnoses are fasciitis (or Shulman's syndrome), eosinophilia-myalgia syndrome, amyloidosis, and scleromyxedema. However, sclerosis is also a sign of POEMS syndrome, carcinoid syndrome, and graft-versus-host reaction. Exogenous and toxic causes of sclerosis should not be omitted: toxic oil, silica, cocaine, L-tryptophane, etc. Localized sclerosis can reveal the presence of morpheiform basal cell carcinoma or scirrhous carcinoma.

Common

Sclerotic scar

D. Lipsker, *Clinical Examination and Differential Diagnosis of Skin Lesions*,
DOI 10.1007/978-2-8178-0411-8_40, © Springer-Verlag France 2013

Table 40.1 Rare causes of systemic sclerosis in newborns and infants

Mucopolysaccharidoses	Hunter: focal sclerosis, contractures, associated neurological and skeletal abnormalities
	Hurler: focal sclerosis, contractures, associated neurological and skeletal abnormalities
	Scheie: focal sclerosis, contractures, associated neurological and skeletal abnormalities
Lysosomal disorders	Neonatal mucolipidosis II (I-cell disease): contractures, thickened skin, facial dysmorphology, psychomotor retardation, organomegaly, skeletal dysplasia
	Farber lipogranulomatosis: contractures, deep-seated plaques and nodules, joint swelling, hoarseness, neurological abnormalities, visceral involvement, malnutrition
Others	Infantile systemic hyalinosis: diffuse thickening of the skin, contractures, gingival hyperplasia, circumoral and rectal papulonodules, stunted growth (mutation capillary morphogenesis factor-2 gene)
	Juvenile hyaline fibromatosis: contractures, deep-seated nodules, gingival hyperplasia, osteolytic lesions (mutation capillary morphogenesis factor-2 gene)
Others	Stiff skin syndrome: similar to deep-seated morphea; rock-hard indurations of the skin accompanied by contractures and discreet hypertrichosis; from a histopathologic point of view, it is a slightly or noninflammatory sclerosis
	Restrictive dermopathy: tight skin, contractures, dysmorphologic face, "O"-shaped open mouth, polyhydramnios, pulmonary hypoplasia, biopsy shows a thick epidermis and a thin dermis; mutations in lamin A or ZMPSTE24
	Hutchinson-Gilford progeria syndrome: sclerotic white macules and plaques or sclerodermoid thickening of the skin, lipoatrophy, prominent veins, pigmentary disorders, alopecia, midfacial "cyanosis," bird face, small stature, skeletal hypoplasia and dysplasia, lamin A mutation
	Geleophysic dysplasia: thickened skin (doughy), contractures, small hands and feet, valvular heart disease, hepatomegaly, bone dysplasia
	Winchester syndrome: contractures, thickening of the skin (with a leather-like consistency), hypertrichosis, autosomal recessive transmission, small stature, corneal opacities, gargoyle face, gingival enlargement, osteoporosis, progressive carpal and tarsal osteolysis, cortical bone thinning, extensive joint damage
	Sclerema neonatorum: generalized sclerosis, poor prognosis
	Parana hard skin syndrome: very stiff skin binding the joints; affects the entire body except eyelids, back of the neck, and ear; restrictive lung disease, death
	Extra-abdominal desmoid tumor (desmoid fibromatosis): shoulders and pelvic girdle, progressively spreading plaques, local malignancy with possible infiltration of muscle and bone
	Subcutaneous fat necrosis of the newborn

Scaling

Desquamation (or scaling) is usually physiological and non-visible and corresponds to normal shedding of epidermal cell residues from the stratum corneum (nonviable cells). It sometimes becomes apparent with the formation of easily detachable scales, unlike keratosis which is firmly adherent. Scaling indicates an epidermal involvement in the pathological process. It can be present either initially or immediately after the onset of a disorder, thus being one of the primary lesions characterizing the disorder. Examples are the scaly erythematous plaques occurring in psoriasis or the scaling which always quickly accompanies erythroderma. It can also occur secondarily, such as with most drug-induced and viral exanthems. Scaly erythematous lesions are particularly common.

Certain types of scaling are specific and may highlight certain mechanisms and/or diseases. For example, shredding (scarlatiniform scales) indicates a brutal interruption of the stratum corneum production, which is typical of superantigen-mediated diseases. Collarette scaling is clinically char-acterized by a scale which is adherent in the periphery but detachable at its center, thus realizing a collarette. It is typical of pityriasis rosea (of Gibert) but also occurs in candidiasis, glucagonoma syndrome, Sneddon-Wilkinson disease, or superficial pemphigus. In psoriasis, scratching with a Brocq's curette will initially reveal white powdered scales ("signe de la tache de bougie" in French terminology), followed by the "sign of the last removable scale" ("le signe de la dernière pellicule détachable" in French terminology), i.e., the thin suprapapillary scales being detached by the curette, and finally the Auspitz sign ("signe de la rosée sanglante" in French terminology), i.e., the formation of bleeding spots due to exposition of the hypervascularized dermal papillae. In pityriasis lichenoides, the primary lesion is an elevated pink or red papule, which rapidly turns brownish-red and is covered with dry, gray, and adherent scales. The lesion then becomes depressed, turning into a macule that retains a scale at its surface. That scale is detachable in one piece using a curette, which is typical of this disorder.

Table 41.1 Main types of scaling with some examples of associated disorders

Shredding	Drug eruption
	Kawasaki disease
	Leptospirosis
	Recurrent perineal erythema
	Recurring scarlatiniform scaled erythema Féréol-Besnier
	Scarlet fever (or scarlatina)
	Staphylococcal toxic shock syndrome
Collarette-like	Candidiasis
	Necrolytic migratory erythema (glucagonoma, enteropathic acrodermatitis, and related diseases)
	Pityriasis rosea (of Gibert)
	Subcorneal pustulosis of Sneddon-Wilkinson
	Superficial pemphigus
Pityriasiform/furfuraceous	Most scaly erythematous diseases
	Mycoses should be kept in mind and mycological examinations performed on a regular basis
Ichthyosiform/scaly	Characteristic of congenital and acquired ichthyoses

D. Lipsker, *Clinical Examination and Differential Diagnosis of Skin Lesions*,
DOI 10.1007/978-2-8178-0411-8_41, © Springer-Verlag France 2013

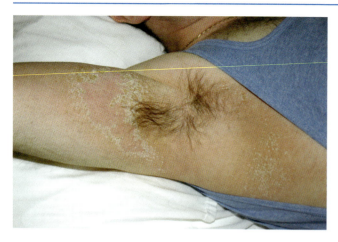

Fig. 41.1 Superficial scaling, relatively thin. Appearance following AGEP (cf. Fig. 14.21)

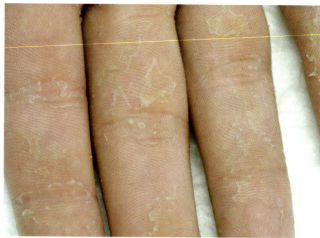

Fig. 41.4 Superficial scaling of the palms. Recurrent palmar peeling ("desquamation estivale en aire"), probably a minor form of dyshidrosis

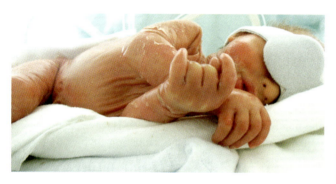

Fig. 41.2 Collodion membrane. Lamellar ichthyosis. The skin is wrapped in a collodion-like membrane, which can sometimes cause constriction, particularly when located around the extremities. This is a syndromic entity as several disorders, for instance, many ichthyoses, can display this type of manifestation

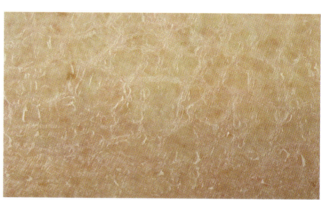

Fig. 41.5 Polygonal scales and eczema craquelé. Statin-induced ichthyosis

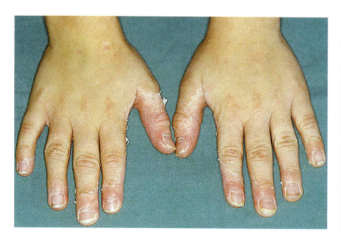

Fig. 41.3 Scaling of fingertips and toes ("en doigt de gants" in French terminology). Recurrent perineal erythema, a variant of the recurring scarlatiniform scaled erythema of Féréol-Besnier

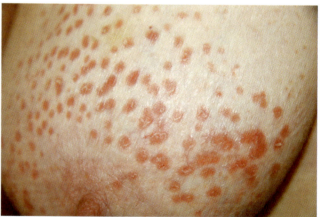

Fig. 41.6 Patchy scale. Pityriasis lichenoides. *Red* macules that retain a scale at their surface. That scale comes off in one piece using a curette, which is typical of this disorder ("squame en pain à cacheter" in French terminology)

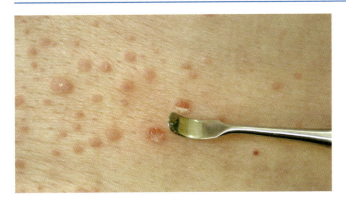

Fig. 41.7 "One piece scaling." Lichen planus. Erythematous papules: only gentle scraping using a Brocq's curette can reveal a scale that comes off in one piece. This illustrates the fact that lichen planus is indeed a dermo-epidermal disorder

These lesions are the consequence of a loss of substance that can either be superficial (erosion), allowing full healing, or deep (ulceration), leaving a scar after healing.

Lesions can be primitive, i.e., the loss of substance is not caused by the evolution of a preexisting lesion; the best example of this type of situation is a posttraumatic ulceration. Otherwise, they can be secondary to other lesions that should be looked for and identified, e.g., the rupture of a bulla or a tumor evolving towards ulceration.

Although leg ulcers are commonplace in elderly people, an isolated ulceration located elsewhere on the integument is never trivial. If a clinical diagnosis cannot be established, biopsy becomes mandatory.

Some ulcerations such as in pyoderma gangrenosum or in hypertensive leg ulcer, as well as those resulting from peripheral arterial disease (limb ischemia), are very painful.

Finally, in immunosuppressed individuals, any type of ulceration should be considered as a manifestation of sepsis, until proven otherwise. The causes of these septic ulcerations are numerous, i.e., bacterial, fungal, and viral. The clinical onset can be violent in patients with neutropenia, e.g., in ecthyma gangrenosum caused by *Pseudomonas aeruginosa*. It can also be insidious, as in certain infections related to atypical mycobacteria. The main causes of leg and mouth ulcers are listed in Boxes 42.1 and 42.2, respectively.

Table 42.1 Main causes of erosions and ulcerations

Type of lesion	Main causes
Erosion	AEC syndrome (eroded scalp skin)
	Candidiasis (intertrigo, balanitis, vulvitis)
	IgA pemphigus and subcorneal pustulosis of Sneddon-Wilkinson
	Impetigo
	Necrolytic migratory erythema (glucagonoma syndrome, enteropathic acrodermatitis, and related disorders)
	Pemphigus
	Staphylococcal scalded skin syndrome
	Toxic epidermal necrolysis
	Traumas and excoriations (caused by scratching)
	Post-vesicular or post-bullous lesions

(continued)

D. Lipsker, *Clinical Examination and Differential Diagnosis of Skin Lesions*,
DOI 10.1007/978-2-8178-0411-8_42, © Springer-Verlag France 2013

Table 42.1 (continued)

Type of lesion	Main causes
Ulcerations	Aplasia cutis congenita
	Bart's syndrome
	Cutaneous Crohn's disease
	Cutaneous dental sinus (dental fistula)
	Cutaneous ulcers (e.g., in Behçet's disease)
	Dermatomyositis
	Drugs (hydroxyurea, methotrexate, etc.)
	Eschar and decubitus ulcer
	Factitial causes
	Fistulated malformation cyst
	Fistulated panniculitis (cytophagic histiocytic panniculitis, fistulating gumma, etc.)
	Focal dermal hypoplasia
	Hemoglobinopathy (particularly sickle-cell anemia)
	Hypertensive leg ulcers (of Martorell)
	Infectious diseases:
	Actinomycosis, nocardiosis (fistula)
	During septicemia (ecthyma gangrenosum, candidiasis, etc.)
	Fungal infection (blastomycosis, sporotrichosis, etc.)
	Herpes virus infections (particularly in immunosuppressed individuals)
	Mycobacterial infection (particularly *M. marinum* and *M. ulcerans*)
	Protozoal infections (leishmaniasis, amebiasis, etc.)
	Pyodermas (ecthyma, anthrax, etc.) and other bacterial infections such as inoculation diseases (tularemia, *Bacillus anthracis*, diphtheria, trypanosomiasis, etc.)
	Sexually transmitted infections (syphilis, chancroid, donovanosis (or granuloma inguinale), etc.)
	Keratoacanthoma
	Lymphomatoid papulosis
	Malacoplakia
	Neurotrophic ulceration
	Painful ear nodule
	Peripheral arterial disease
	Pyoderma gangrenosum
	Shooter's patch: chronic ulceration at the site of heroin injection
	Snake and spider bite
	Traumas
	Ulcerated cutaneous lymphoma
	Ulcerated tumors (squamous cell carcinomas, basal cell carcinomas, etc.)
	Ulcers caused by vasculitis (granulomatosis with polyangiitis, temporal arteritis, PAN, Churg-Strauss syndrome, etc.) and thrombosis (AAS, angioendotheliomatosis, etc.)
	Venous ulcer

PAN polyarteritis nodosa, *AAS* antiphospholipid antibody syndrome

Erosion

An erosion is often the late manifestation of a ruptured bulla.

Extended erosion can be observed in toxic epidermal necrolysis and staphylococcal scalded skin syndrome. A glucagonoma syndrome and acrodermatitis enteropathica must be suspected, particularly when the erosions spread outside the folds.

Ulceration

An isolated ulceration is always suspect of being a tumor (carcinoma, melanoma, lymphoma, etc.).

Other causes of ulcerations are infections, such as in septicemias caused by infection with *Pseudomonas* (ecthyma gangrenosum) and *Candida*, or in primarily cutaneous disorders ("inoculation chancre": syphilis, tularemia, diphtheria, *Bacillus anthracis*, and late pyodermas), or the result of a gummatous fistulization and/or evolution (caused by mycobacteria, blastomycosis, and actinomycosis). Vasculitic and thrombotic ulcers, as well as ulcerated gumma in cytophagic histiocytic panniculitis, should be kept in mind.

Common

Bullous or exogenous erosions are common. Impetigo, herpes, and candidiasis are common, as well as traumatic ulcers and vascular-nervous trophic disorders. Neoplastic ulcers are common in the elderly.

Box 42.1 Main Causes of Leg Ulcers

Venous insufficiency
  Primary, secondary (postthrombotic), atrophie blanche
Peripheral arterial disease and microangiopathy
  Arterial hypertension, obstructive arteriopathies, arterial embolisms, cholesterol embolisms, livedoid vasculitis, arteriovenous fistulas
Vasculitis
  Primary (PAN, etc.) and secondary (mixed connective tissue disease, etc.)
Blood disorders
  Fibrinolytic disorders and hypercoagulability
  Protein C or S deficiency, activated protein C resistance, hemolytic anemias (sickle-cell anemia, thalassemia, spherocytosis), myeloproliferative syndrome (myelodysplastic, thrombocythemia, polycythemia), lymphoproliferative syndrome (multiple myelomas and Waldenström's macroglobulinemia)
Neuropathies
  Amyloidoses, paraplegia (spinal cord injury in L1), poliomyelitis, peripheral nerve injury (diabetes, leprosy, traumas), etc.
Infections
  Osteomyelitis, ecthyma, pyoderma caused by infection with *Pseudomonas aeruginosa*, ulcers caused by infection with *Pasteurella multocida*, tropical ulcers, mycobacterial infections (tuberculosis, leprosy, Buruli ulcer), diphtheria, tularemia, cat scratch disease, treponematoses (endemic, syphilis), deep-seated mycoses, parasitoses (leishmaniasis, guinea worm, filarioses, etc.)
Traumas
  Bites; insect bites; physical, chemical, or thermal traumas; pathomimesis
Dermatological disorders
  Pyoderma gangrenosum, necrobiosis lipoidica, autoimmune bullous diseases, systemic sclerosis, erythema induratum of Bazin, sarcoidosis, chilblain, panniculitis, halogenodermas, radiodermatitis, pathomimesis

Tumors
  Carcinomas (basal cell carcinoma, squamous cell carcinoma, verrucous carcinoma), melanoma, Kaposi's sarcoma, lymphomas, metastases, etc.
Miscellaneous
  Chromosomal anomalies (Klinefelter, Werner), prolidase deficiency, chronic renal insufficiency, hyperparathyroidism, calcinoses, gout, and hydroxyurea chemotherapy

Box 42.2 Main Causes of Ulcerations of the Oral Mucosa

Agranulocytosis, cyclic neutropenia and blood disorders
Bednar's aphthae in neonates
Blastomycosis
Carcinoma
Dermatopolymyositis
Drugs: methotrexate, nicorandil, NSAID (nonsteroidal anti-inflammatory drugs), etc.
Epidermolysis bullosa
Erosive stomatitis associated with antinuclear antibodies
Erythema multiforme
Hemorrhagic bullous stomatitis
Histiocytosis
Histoplasmosis
HIV infection (and opportunistic infections such as histoplasmosis, blastomycosis, paracoccidioidomycosis, and cryptococcosis)
Infection caused by *Herpesviridae* (simplex, zoster, CMV, EBV, etc.)
Inflammatory bowel diseases (aphthae, erosions, pyostomatitis vegetans)
Laryngo-onycho-cutaneous syndrome (AR, LAMA3 gene): granulation tissue of the skin, nails, and mucosa
Lichen planus
Ligneous gingivitis and conjunctivitis associated with plasminogen deficiency
Lupus erythematosus and other connective tissue diseases
Lymphoma
Mechanical causes (including Riga-Fede disease)
Mouth ulcers (simple, giant oral ulcer or Sutton's ulcer, herpetiform) and their causes
Paracoccidioidomycosis
Pemphigus, pemphigoid, and other autoimmune bullous dermatoses
Primary syphilis
Severe combined immune deficiency (SCID)
Stevens-Johnson syndrome
Toxin-mediated and chemically mediated diseases
Tuberculosis

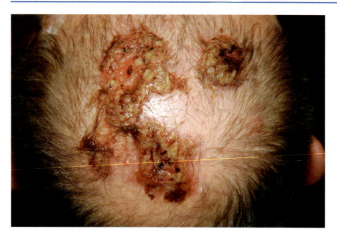

Fig. 42.1 Pustular and crusted erosions. Erosive pustular dermatosis of the scalp

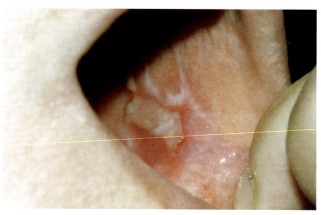

Fig. 42.3 Fibrinous ulcer in the jugal mucosa. Erosive lichen planus. Note the peripheral erythroleukokeratosis

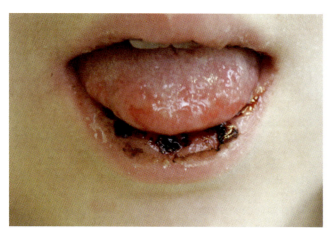

Fig. 42.2 Hemorrhagic crusted eroded lips. Erythema multiforme

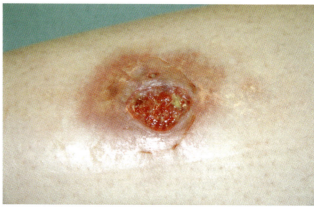

Fig. 42.4 Leg ulcer. Necrobiosis lipoidica. Note the area surrounding the ulcer, which is erythematous, atrophic, and telangiectatic

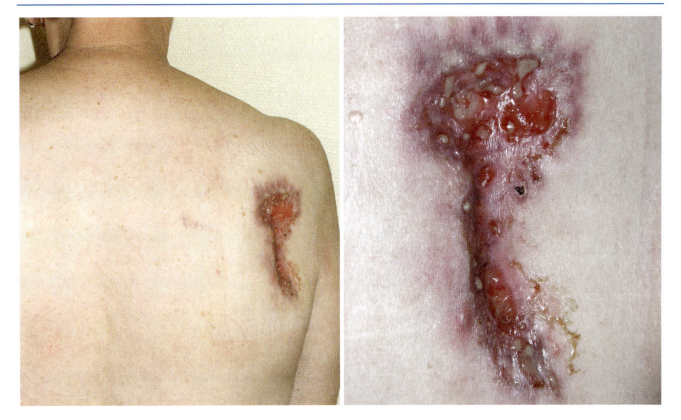

Fig. 42.5 Chronic skin ulcer. Granulomatosis with polyangiitis. Note the purulent periphery; chronic skin ulcer in granulomatosis with polyangiitis may have the appearance of pyoderma gangrenosum (cf. Figs. 15.43, 15.44, and 15.45)

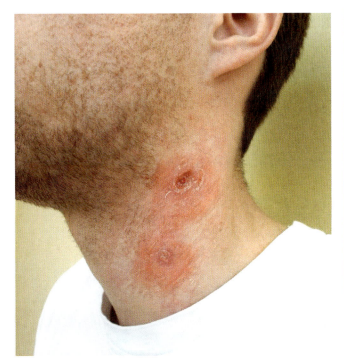

Fig. 42.6 Crusted ulcers of the neck. Leishmaniasis

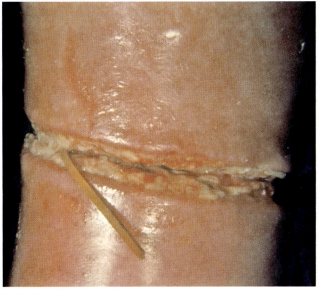

Fig. 42.7 Circumferential ulcer caused by an elastic band. Constant pressure may lead to ulceration through complex mechanisms (such as physical pressure, maceration, and ischemia)

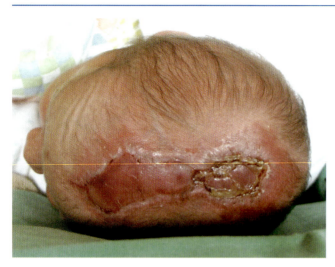

Fig. 42.8 Aplasia cutis of the vertex. This localized absence of skin leads to a scarring linear cutaneous depression on the vertex. This type of congenital anomaly can be isolated or be the marker of dysraphism. It can also be syndromic (Adams-Oliver syndrome, Johanson-Blizzard syndrome, oculoauriculovertebral syndrome, chromosomal anomalies, etc.)

Necrosis

Necrosis is the consequence of ischemia. It entails insensitivity to all modes, followed by the formation of black and devitalized skin which gradually becomes lined and separated from healthy adjacent skin (by an eliminating groove), in a matter of days. Until proven otherwise, necrosis must always be treated as a medical or surgical emergency. Diagnosis of necrosis at the stage of black necrotic plaque comes too late. Early diagnosis is not always simple and requires experience. The following signs should be noticed: a painless part within a painful area, a pallor or drop in skin temperature within an erythematous area, and particularly a purpura with dark coloration. A needle can be used (SC or IM) to prick the suspected areas. In the absence of neuropathy, painlessness indicates a serious situation. The removal of the needle induces bleeding. If not, the necrosis is evolutive. It is therefore imperative to determine its cause, and appropriate treatment must be implemented without delay. The onset of necrosis can either reflect the severity of a cutaneous disorder (e.g., infectious cellulitis) or represent the cutaneous manifestation of a serious systemic disease (such as DIC, calciphylaxis).

The clinical context, the extension of the necrosis, and the associated signs are essential for establishing diagnosis (e.g., in the presence of localized necrosis in an immunosuppressed patient or a patient with diabetic acidoketosis, a mucormycosis must be suspected, first and foremost).

Table 43.1 Main causes of necroses

Mechanism	Main causes
Non-thrombotic vascular obstructions	Acute ischemia
	Buerger's disease
	Calciphylaxis
	Compressive hematoma
	Embolisms (i.e., cardiac, or caused by cholesterol crystals, or fat)
	Ergotism and drugs (dihydroergotamine + macrolides, vasopressors, bleomycin, etc.)
	Hypertensive leg ulcer
	Peripheral arterial disease
	Phlegmasia cerulea
	Pseudoxanthoma elasticum
	Vascular dissection and direct arterial injury
	Vascular type of acrokeratosis paraneoplastica
	Vasculitis (PAN, granulomatosis with polyangiitis, necrotizing leukocytoclastic vasculitis, etc.)
Vascular thromboses	Anticoagulant-induced necrosis
	Blood disorders (polycythemia, thrombocythemia, etc.)
	Catastrophic antiphospholipid syndrome and APLS
	Cryoproteins (cryofibrinogenemia, cold agglutinins, etc.)
	Deficiency of coagulation proteins
	DIC (in patients with meningococcal purpura fulminans, Gram septicemia, etc.)
	Paraproteinemia (myeloma, Waldenström's disease, monoclonal cryoglobulinemia, etc.)
	Reactive angioendotheliomatoses
	Thalassemia, sickle-cell anemia

(continued)

D. Lipsker, *Clinical Examination and Differential Diagnosis of Skin Lesions*, DOI 10.1007/978-2-8178-0411-8_43, © Springer-Verlag France 2013

Table 43.1 (continued)

Mechanism	Main causes
Infections	Ecthyma gangrenosum
	Meningococcemia
	Miscellaneous, particularly in immunosuppressed patients: zoster and varicella, aspergillosis, mucormycosis, *Bacillus anthracis*, amebiasis, noma, diphtheria, syphilis, rickettsioses, *Stenotrophomonas maltophilia*, etc.
	Necrotizing fasciitis and other infectious cellulitis (Fournier, gas gangrene, etc.)
Physical agents	Burns (thermal, electrical, chemical, X-rays, etc.)
	Frostbite
	Mechanical trauma
Iatrogenic and toxin-mediated	Anticoagulants (coumarin necrosis)
	Bleomycin
	Chemotherapy extravasation injury, arterial cannulation, etc.
	Digital pulse oximeter used for intensive care patients
	Ergotism
	Intradermal or hypodermal injection of deconditioned substances (e.g., buprenorphine, acetaminophen)
	Nicolau's livedoid dermatitis (by accidental intra-arterial injection)
	Snake and spider bite
	Vasoconstrictors (adrenalin, dopamine, etc.)
Other	Acute necrotizing ulcerative pityriasis lichenoides

PAN polyarteritis nodosa, *DIC* disseminated intravascular coagulation, *APLS* antiphospholipid syndrome

Do Not Miss

A cutaneous necrosis is always an emergency. It usually indicates a progressive ischemia. It is observed in serious infections (necrotizing fasciitis, meningococcemia, septicemia, ecthyma gangrenosum, *Bacillus anthracis* infection, rickettsioses, opportunistic infections [mucormycosis, aspergillosis]), as well as in "common" infections in debilitated patients (varicella, zoster, syphilis). It can also reflect a vascular obstruction that can be non-thrombotic (peripheral arterial disease, emboli, dissection, vasculitis, compression, PXE, calciphylaxis) or thrombotic (DIC, catastrophic APLS, hereditary thrombophilia, protein precipitation, etc.).

It can also be caused by external factors such as irradiation or toxic substances (e.g., snake bite, high doses of vasoconstrictors, coumarin necrosis)

Common

Caustic and exogenous causes of necrosis (burns, frostbite, trauma, compressive hematoma) are the most common. Martorell's hypertensive leg ulcer, necrotizing evolution of erysipela in the context of diabetes, or limb ischemia. Digital necroses occur in intensive care, following the use of vasomotor drugs and/or pulse oximeters.

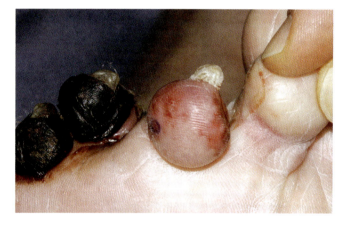

Fig. 43.1 Toe necrosis. Atheroembolism. Note the discreet reticulate purpura on the tip of the third toe

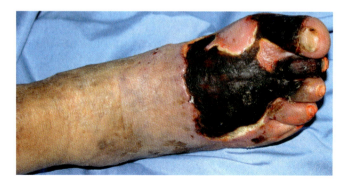

Fig. 43.2 Necrosis. Erysipela. In a patient with peripheral arterial disease and/or diabetes, decompensation of a latent microangiopathy or macroangiopathy may be induced by erysipela. Distal necrosis then occurs, which is however not an indication for cellulitis surgery, but eventually for an emergency revascularization surgery, if possible

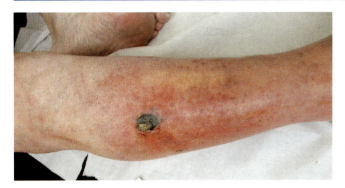

Fig. 43.3 Leg necrosis surrounded by erythema. *Pasteurella* infection

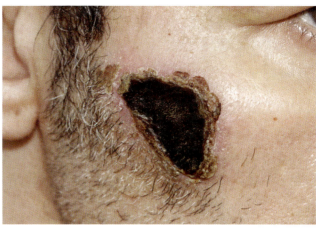

Fig. 43.5 Jugal necrosis. Eschar. This eschar is caused by prolonged vascular compression, in a patient with psychosis and clinophilia

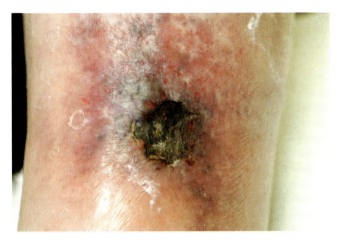

Fig. 43.4 Livedoid erythema with central necrosis. Hypertensive leg ulcer

Index

Page numbers in italics refer to photographs. Page numbers in bold refer to the most important occurrence.

D. Lipsker, *Clinical Examination and Differential Diagnosis of Skin Lesions*,
DOI 10.1007/978-2-8178-0411-8, © Springer-Verlag France 2013